Victoria Wills

KETOGENIC
DIET FOR WOMEN AFTER 50

*The Complete Guide to Success on the Keto Diet
and 120 Delicious Recipes + 30-Day Keto Meal Plan
to Lose Weight, Heal Your Body and Start Asap*

Table of Contents

INTRODUCTION...........................8

CHAPTER 1: WHAT IS KETO? 12

IS GOING KETO ALRIGHT FOR PEOPLE
WITH DIABETES?..........................12
HOW THE BODY CHANGES WHEN
YOU'RE OVER 50...........................13
WHY SHOULD YOU SWITCH TO KETO?
....13

CHAPTER 2: WHAT DOES A
KETOGENIC DIET MEAN FOR A
WOMEN AFTER 50?...................14

BODY CHANGES AFTER 50, WHAT
CHANGES IN THE WOMEN'S BODY? .14

CHAPTER 3: BENEFITS OF THE KETO
DIET FOR WOMAN AFTER 50 16

REDUCTION OF CRAVINGS AND
APPETITE 16
REDUCTION OF RISK OF HEART DISEASE
....16
REDUCES CHANCES OF HAVING HIGH
BLOOD PRESSURE 16
FIGHTS TYPE 2 DIABETES................17
INCREASES THE PRODUCTION OF HDL
....17
SUPPRESSES YOUR APPETITE 17
CHANGES IN CHOLESTEROL LEVELS...17
INCREASE BODY ENERGY LEVEL 18
BOOST BRAIN FUNCTION AND MENTAL
CLARITY 18
SLOWING DOWN AGING PROCESS ...18
REDUCE INFLAMMATION 19

CHAPTER 4: PRACTICAL TIPS FOR
SUCCESS 20

START BUILDING ON IMMUNITY 20
CONSIDER QUITTING SMOKING.......20
STAY SOCIAL 21
HEALTH SCREENINGS YOU SHOULD GET
AFTER YOUR FIFTIES 21

CHAPTER 5: HOW DOES KETO DIET
WORKS? 24

SIGNS THAT YOU ARE IN KETOSIS 26

CHAPTER 6: COMMON MISTAKES
....28

EXCESS PROTEIN 28
EXCESS NUTS AND DAIRY..............28
ADAPTION TIME...........................29
EXCESS CARBOHYDRATES 29
SNACKING...................................29
DEHYDRATION AND ELECTROLYTES ..29
MINDSET.....................................30

CHAPTER 7: RECOMMENDED KETO
FOODS......................................32

FOOD ALLOWED IN UNLIMITED
QUANTITIES 32
FOODS AUTHORIZED IN MODERATE
QUANTITIES 34

CHAPTER 8: FOOD AND BEVERAGE
TO AVOID 36

BREAD AND GRAINS.....................36
FRUITS 36
VEGETABLES...............................36
PASTA..36

CEREAL 36

BEER 37

SWEETENED YOGURT 37

JUICE 37

LOW-FAT AND FAT-FREE SALAD
DRESSINGS................................... 37

BEANS AND LEGUMES 37

SUGAR 37

CHIPS AND CRACKERS 37

MILK 38

GLUTEN-FREE BAKED GOODS 38

**CHAPTER 9: MORE ABOUT KETO
DIET 40**

HORMONE BALANCE..................... 40

MENOPAUSE 40

AUTOPHAGY 42

CHAPTER 10: BREAKFAST 44

1. BREAKFAST OMELETTE WITH
MUSHROOMS............................. 45

2. MORNING COCONUT PORRIDGE
.... 46

3. DAIRY-FREE PIZZA 47

4. SESAME KETO BAGELS 48

5. BAKED EGGS IN AVOCADO
HALVES 49

6. SPICY CREAM CHEESE PANCAKES
.... 50

7. BRACING GINGER SMOOTHIE 51

8. MORNING COFFEE WITH CREAM
.... 51

9. CHEESY BREAKFAST MUFFINS 52

10. SPINACH, MUSHROOM, AND
GOAT CHEESE FRITTATA 53

11. CHEESY BROCCOLI MUFFINS . 54

12. BERRY CHOCOLATE BREAKFAST
BOWL 55

13. "COCO-NUT" GRANOLA.......56

CHAPTER 11: LUNCH...................58

14. CHEESY CHICKEN CAULIFLOWER
....59

15. CHICKEN SOUP 60

16. CHICKEN AVOCADO SALAD....61

17. CHICKEN BROCCOLI DINNER ..62

18. LEMON BAKED SALMON 63

19. CAULIFLOWER MASH 64

20. BAKED SALMON..................65

21. SLOW COOKER CHILLI 66

CHAPTER 12: DINNER 68

22. BEEF-STUFFED MUSHROOMS 69

23. RIB ROAST 70

24. BEEF STIR FRY 71

25. GRILLED PORK WITH SALSA ...72

26. CHICKEN PESTO 73

27. GARLIC PARMESAN CHICKEN
WINGS 74

28. CRISPY BAKED SHRIMP 75

29. HERBED MEDITERRANEAN FISH
FILLET 76

30. MUSHROOM STUFFED WITH
RICOTTA 77

31. THAI CHOPPED SALAD..........78

32. CHICKEN KURMA................79

33. GREEN CHICKEN CURRY........80

34. BEEF WITH BELL PEPPERS 81

CHAPTER 13: POULTRY RECIPES..82

35. EGG BUTTER 83

36. SHREDDED CHICKEN IN A
LETTUCE WRAP 84

37. BACON-WRAPPED CHICKEN
BITES 85

38.   CHEESY BACON WRAPPED
CHICKEN 86
39.   BEANS AND SAUSAGE..........87
40.   PAPRIKA RUBBED CHICKEN....88
41.   TERIYAKI CHICKEN 89
42.   CHILI LIME CHICKEN WITH
COLESLAW 90
43.   LIME GARLIC CHICKEN THIGHS
....91
44.   BACON RANCH DEVILED EGGS
....92
45.   DEVILED EGGS WITH
MUSHROOMS 93
46.   CHICKEN AND PEANUT STIR-FRY
....94
47.   LEMONY CHICKEN DRUMSTICKS
....95
48.   LEMONY CHICKEN THIGHS 96
49.   TURKEY MEATLOAF 97

CHAPTER 14: MEAT RECIPES....... 98

50.   BEEF AND BROCCOLI STIR-FRY
....99
51.   ROSEMARY ROASTED PORK
WITH CAULIFLOWER 100
52.   SWEET & SOUR PORK 101
53.   GARLIC PORK LOIN 101
54.   KETO GRILLED LAMB STEAKS
....102
55.   STEAK WITH PESTO...........103
56.   HERBED LAMB CHOPS........104
57.   GRILLED PORK CHOPS 105

CHAPTER 15: SEAFOOD & FISH
RECIPES.................................. 106

58.   CRAB SALAD....................107
59.   EASY SEAFOOD SALAD........108
60.   EASY CRAB CAKES 109

61.   NUTRITIOUS TUNA PATTIES 110
62.   QUICK BUTTER COD 111
63.   BAKED TILAPIA 112
64.   SHRIMP AVOCADO SALAD .. 113
65.   PAPRIKA SHRIMP 114
66.   ZINGY LEMON FISH 115
67.   KETO THAI FISH WITH CURRY
AND COCONUT 116
68.   CREAMY MACKEREL 117
69.   LIME MACKEREL..............118
70.   TURMERIC TILAPIA 118
71.   WALNUT SALMON MIX......119

CHAPTER 16: SALAD RECIPES 120

72.   BACON AVOCADO SALAD ... 121
73.   CAULIFLOWER AND CASHEW
NUT SALAD 122
74.   SALMON AND LETTUCE SALAD
....123
75.   PRAWNS SALAD WITH MIXED
LETTUCE GREENS 124
76.   SHRIMP, TOMATO, AND
AVOCADO SALAD 125

CHAPTER 17: SOUP AND STEWS126

77.   HEARTY FALL STEW...........127
78.   CHICKEN MUSHROOM SOUP
....128
79.   COLD GREEN BEANS AND
AVOCADO SOUP 129
80.   CREAMY MIXED SEAFOOD SOUP
....130
81.   ROASTED TOMATO AND
CHEDDAR SOUP 131
82.   HEALTHY CELERY SOUP 132
83.   COCONUT CURRY CAULIFLOWER
SOUP 133

84. NUTMEG PUMPKIN SOUP... 134

85. THAI COCONUT VEGETABLE SOUP 135

CHAPTER 18: DESSERT RECIPES 136

86. PUMPKIN SPICED ALMONDS 137

87. COCO-MACADAMIA FAT BOMBS 138

88. TZATZIKI DIP WITH CAULIFLOWER 139

89. CURRY-ROASTED MACADAMIA NUTS 140

90. SESAME ALMOND FAT BOMBS 141

91. COCONUT CHIA PUDDING .. 141

92. ORANGE LIME PUDDING 142

93. ALMOND COCOA SPREAD... 143

CHAPTER 19: CONDIMENTS, SAUCES AND SPREADS 144

94. TACO SEASONING 144

95. PUMPKIN PIE SPICE.......... 145

96. GARAM MASALA POWDER . 146

97. POULTRY SEASONING 147

98. YOGURT TZATZIKI 148

99. BASIL PESTO 149

100. ALMOND BUTTER 150

101. LEMON CURD SPREAD .. 151

102. TAHINI SPREAD........... 152

CHAPTER 20: BEVERAGE AND SMOOTHIES 154

103. COCONUT SMOOTHIE ... 155

104. ALMOND SMOOTHIE 155

105. SUMMER BERRY SMOOTHIE 156

106. FRUITY PARSLEY SMOOTHIE 156

107. LEMONY SMOOTHIE......157

108. ORANGE, CARROT & KALE SMOOTHIE 157

109. CREAMY STRAWBERRY & CHERRY SMOOTHIE 158

110. LIME AND GINGER GREEN SMOOTHIE 158

111. STRAWBERRY SPINACH SMOOTHIE 159

112. MANGO & ROCKET ARUGULA SMOOTHIE 159

CHAPTER 21: SNACKS 160

113. FRIED GREEN BEANS ROSEMARY 161

114. CHEESY CAULIFLOWER CROQUETTES 161

115. CHEESY MUSHROOM SLICES 162

116. ASPARAGUS FRIES 163

117. KALE CHIPS 164

118. GUACAMOLE 164

119. ZUCCHINI NOODLES 165

120. CAULIFLOWER SOUFFLÉ .166

CHAPTER 22: A COMPLETE 30-DAY MEAL PLAN WITH WEEKLY MENU 168

WEEK 1 168

WEEK 2 169

WEEK 3 170

WEEK 4 171

CONCLUSION..........................172

Introduction

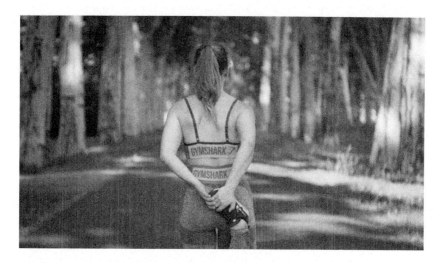

A re you a middle-aged woman that needs health advice? Do you feel helpless about your weight and are worried about illnesses? Are you looking for a diet that is suitable for you? Then this book might be just what you need!

This diet is a popular discussion in general media. However, they claim that it's only good for weight loss. This is the wrong way of thinking. Each person is unique; they have their own levels of activity, appetite, and eating habits. You might have heard about these factors, as they are well known. According to a person's lifestyle, the metabolic rates of individuals differ from each other. One such factor affects weight loss, dieting, and hunger that has not been mentioned: hormonal discrepancy or differences in hormone levels.

Activities in our body interact with each other and coordinate certain changes with different chemical messengers. A major portion that carries this out is endocrine hormones. These chemicals are released in our blood and carry a signal that produces specific actions. Women have different sex hormones, namely estrogen and progesterone.

These sex hormones are released by ovaries; they fluctuate and elevate, along with our menstrual cycle. But, as a woman ages, these levels decline and then stay that way after menopause occurs.

One aging sign for women is when their menstrual cycle ceases permanently. This occurs around the age of 50, and it is called menopause. The time before this occurs is known as perimenopause. You will know that menopause is near when you start noticing irregularities in your cycle and flow. This not only affects the reproductive system but also has profound changes in a woman's body. You will know that menopause has occurred when you have reached the near 50s and stopped having periods for over a year. If you bleed after one year has passed, then it is advised that you get that checked as quickly as you can.

The most noticeable and significant effect of menopause is that our ovaries stop releasing eggs or ovaries. This means we can no longer get pregnant and conceive. Because ovaries have stopped their function, they don't release estrogen or progesterone anymore. The decline of these hormones results in many changes as well.

The changes you will notice will happen gradually. Headaches, hot flashes, and problems with sleep are some of the symptoms. You will become moody and more irritable. Your breasts will shrink in size, and you'll have a lower libido. You will have to go to the bathroom more often because of the increased frequency of urination. Vaginal tissue and pubic muscle tones will also significantly decrease, and you will have a greater chance of yeast infections and irritation. You will start having weak bones, and you will be at a higher risk for osteoporosis. This occurs because not only do estrogen levels decrease but also, because of old age, growth hormones also decrease. Both have a role in bone remodeling, which puts a woman at a higher risk for this disease.

Hormones determine to some extent, where and how much fat is stored throughout the body. A bit of a noticeable change will occur between pre- and post-menopause, and your body will look different. During youth, fats are stored in the hips and breasts; post-menopause, it starts being stored in the belly and becomes belly fat. You may be dieting and are eating healthier than you ever have, but because of physiology, you will see your waist disappear. This process makes being healthy and slim a challenge, but it can be done. I am living proof.

You may think that you have to try a completely new diet approach to get you through this phase in life, and you may even think about giving up. If it is the normal process of the body, then it can't be helped.

That is the wrong way to think! After menopause, the importance of your health and diet is more than before. They make things hard, but with a good diet plan, guidelines, and your determination, you can and will lose weight and keep it off.

You may be asking, "Who am I to talk about this subject?" My name is Sandra Grant. I am a woman in my fifties, enjoying my life filled with energy. A couple of years ago, I was overweight. I was doing everything you would think that would've kept my weight down. I was very active, was working five days a week, was cautious of what I ate, and yet my waist accumulated fat. I was pretty distressed, didn't like looking at myself, and was embarrassed in front of my husband. I wanted to change! I started trying out different diets. One after another, they all disappointed me in the end. I got no results. Then, I looked up this trending diet called keto. I wanted only to shed pounds, so I decided to give this one a try, which is the most effective way of losing weight. To my surprise, in a couple of weeks, I saw results. My clothes that were getting tight suddenly became loose and comfortable. I lost a lot of weight in a couple of months. It felt like a dream.

Open your internet browser and search; you will see a new type of diet that is getting all the attention. You will see a young woman talking about her experience and praising the diet. You look for other people's advice on the topic; you will see they have their own opinions, but one thing in common would be that they all will be in their late teens or are young adults. You would rarely see a diet targeting the elderly, even though arguably, this is the group that needs the most attention regarding health. You need to take care of yourself. Even if your problems are not trending, don't overlook them.

It is my passion now to help other women like me achieve their goals without being disappointed. In this book, I will tell you the secret of my success. I will introduce you to this amazing diet that will quickly get you the body you want.

Just a little break to ask you something that means a lot to me:

What Did You Think of Ketogenic Diet for Women after 50?

First of all, thank you for purchasing this book **Ketogenic Diet for Women after 50**. I know you could have picked between a significant number of cookbooks, but you chose this one, and for that, I am incredibly grateful.

I hope it will add value and quality to your everyday life. If it were so, it would be nice if you could share this book with your friends and family by posting on Facebook and Twitter.

If you enjoyed this book and found some benefit in reading this, I'd like to hear from you and hope that you could take some time to post a review on Amazon. Your feedback and support will significantly improve my writing craft for future projects and make this cookbook even better.

If you have purchased the paperback version through Amazon, just going to your purchases section and Click "Write a Review", or if you have purchased it in a library, just going to Amazon and search this book (Title and the Name of the Author) and click "Write a Review".

I want you to know that your review is very important, I will be happy to hear your thoughts about this book.

I wish you all the best in your future success!

Victoria Wills

CHAPTER 1:

What Is Keto?

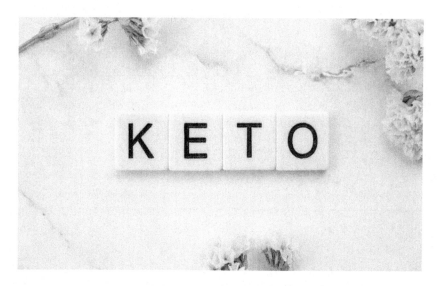

A s you'd probably already know, the ketogenic diet is a low-carb diet where you eliminate or minimize the consumption of carbohydrates. The extra carbs are replaced by proteins and fats while you cut back on pastries and sugar.

Is Going Keto Alright for People With Diabetes?

Now you're probably wondering, what do I do if I have diabetes? For starters, speak to your personal physician.

Talking to your physician is important regardless of what kind of diet you choose. However, note that keto diets generally do work well to improve insulin sensitivity.

For better results, seek a doctor's help if you have diabetes.

Keto diets can have a drastic impact on your body and overall lifestyle; hence it's always better to seek extra guidance from a professional.

How the Body Changes When You're Over 50

This isn't going to be fun to read, but once you hit your 50s, you're likely to experience a number of changes in your body. The most common include:

- Weight Gain

According to the Centers for Disease Control and Prevention (CDC), men and women are likely to gain one to two pounds each year as they transition from adulthood to middle age. This doesn't get any better for women as they hit menopause. While gaining belly fat isn't directly linked to menopause, hormonal changes may cause you to pack a few pounds, depending on lifestyle and environmental changes.

- Metabolism Slows Down

You've probably heard a lot about your metabolism changing as you grow older. That's probably why you can't chow down junk food as you used to when you were in your teens. So, what is metabolism, and how does it affect your body?

In simple terms, metabolism is how quickly your body processes or converts food and liquids into energy. As you grow older, metabolism slows down, and the body starts to convert those extra calories into fat. This is probably why you should skip those convenience meals and start to eat healthier.

Why Should You Switch to Keto?

Once you start to hit 50, you likely don't indulge in strenuous activities anymore, which is why you'll be needing fewer calories to function. This is when you should start eliminating added sugars from your diet. In addition, most packaged meals or meals provided in the hospital for the elderly are processed and contain empty calories, including mashed potatoes, bread, pasta and puddings. Not only do these foods taste bland, but they also lack nutrition to keep your body strong and healthy. Plus, a low-carb diet that is rich in healthy vegetables and meat will prove to be far better for folks suffering from insulin insensitivity and your overall health. Hence, start reading food labels more often and opt for healthier options. A recent study from the Hebrew University of Jerusalem has indicated how eating a diet rich in healthy fats can help you lose weight in the long run.

CHAPTER 2:

What Does a Ketogenic Diet Mean For a Women After 50?

The main thing that should be of more interest to seniors is how to use the ketogenic diet. But your curiosity might move further, and you might want to understand what has changed between you and younger self if you two are into Keto right now.

Well, you are both humans just that age and time has played its part. Unlike before, most of your body system have stopped maturing. So, let's see what has changed and the differences.

The truth remains that aging comes with nutritional challenges. There are different reasons for this, and they can be classified into different categories.

Generally, when we were young, our parents pay close attention to what they give us—their kids—to consume because any mistake can be costly at this stage. But as we age and have more freedom, we consume a lot of things. Then in the middle of our lives, we begin to think that we aren't growing, not like children anymore. You have reached the peak of your height, and such thoughts can be the beginning of unhealthy— and if not unhealthy, unmindful—consumption of food.

Another reason has too much responsibility. If you have a lot of responsibility on your shoulder, you will be more concerned with lifting them than thinking of what you will eat tonight, the following morning, and the day after that. Planning your meal isn't your thing anymore, and cooking is time-consuming at this stage.

Body Changes After 50, What Changes in the Women's Body?

You might have noticed that the metabolism rate slows down as you age. The body generally becomes weaker and weaker. It means our body is prone to the sickness of some sought. A little headache can happen and cause more havoc than before. Some of the chronic diseases common at old age include arthritis, dementia, depression, respiratory diseases, etc. These diseases can affect appetite and what you are asked to consume. It will further contribute to the impairment of the nutritional requirement of the body.

Another reason is the consequences of the nutritional actions of younger years. If you have been consuming a low diet all your life, you might not notice the weight until you are 50, and the whole thing has accumulated. It could affect your teeth or your taste for certain foods. These things could make your nutritional needs change.

The last factor we will be talking about is the natural happenings in the body. With age, the bones will get weaker, and we will likely lose some of our dentition. We will experience a loss of muscle mass as we turn 50, and this will be more evident by the time we clock 60. Now that you have seen the factors that affect our nutritional needs and how it changes, you shouldn't expect your body to respond to food consumption the way it used to be when you were younger.

But the good thing is the number of older adults might surpass that of younger generations in the nearest future. It is possible due to several factors, such as procreation control and improved health services and facilities. But there will also be a kind of burden on the providers of the services and supports.

It will be wise as a person to be interested in your dietary needs and work towards achieving it. That way, it will not be the effort of someone else in the long run, and you will stay healthier and happier for a more extended period, even till death.

Obviously, it is essential for all ages, either 12 or 50, to want to age gracefully. Aging gracefully means aging without serious health issues and concerns. It is a lot of work in this age where there are many temptations—snacks, distractions, ads—that want us to eat unhealthily. That's why many obese people are around and why "loose a million pounds in five days" kind of programs sell these days quickly.

Congratulations, because I know you are not like most people; you take your health seriously. You should reread this guide and get started. You need to know some things about your middle age and Keto's nutritional reaction to your body. There are quite differences between being young and being older.

CHAPTER 3:

Benefits of the Keto Diet for Woman After 50

Reduction of Cravings and Appetite

Many people gain weight simply because they cannot control their cravings and appetite for caloric foods. The ketogenic diet helps eliminate these problems, but it does not mean that you will never be hungry or want to eat. You will feel hungry but only when you have to eat. Several studies have shown that the less carbohydrates you eat, the less you eat overall. Eating healthier foods that are high in fat helps reduce your appetite, as you lose more weight faster on a low-fat diet. The reason for this is that low carbohydrate diets help lower insulin levels, as your body does not need too much insulin to convert glycogen to glucose while eliminating excess water in your body. This diet helps you reduce visceral fat. In this way, you will get a slimmer look and shape. It is the most difficult fat to lose, as it surrounds the organs as it increases. High doses can cause inflammation and insulin resistance. Coconut oil can produce an immediate source of energy as it increases ketone levels in your body.

Reduction of Risk of Heart Disease

Triglycerides, fat molecules in your body, have close links with heart disease. They are directly proportional as the more the number of triglycerides, the higher your chances of suffering from heart disease. You can reduce the number of free triglycerides in your body by reducing the number of carbohydrates, as is in the keto diets.

Reduces Chances of Having High Blood Pressure

Weight loss and blood pressure have a close connection; thus, since you are losing weight while on the keto diet, it will affect your blood pressure.

Fights Type 2 Diabetes

Type two diabetes develops as a result of insulin resistance. This is a result of having huge amounts of glucose in your system, with the keto diet this is not a possibility due to the low carbohydrate intake.

Increases the Production of HDL

High-density lipoprotein is referred to as good cholesterol. It is responsible for caring calories to your liver, thus can be reused. High fat and low carbohydrate diets increase the production of HDL in your body, which also reduces your chances of getting a heart disease. Low-density lipoprotein is referred to as bad cholesterol.

Suppresses Your Appetite

It is a strange but true effect of the keto diet. It was thought that this was a result of the production of ketones, but this was proven wrong as a study taken between people on a regular balanced diet and some on the keto diet and their appetites were generally the same. It, however, helps to suppress appetite as it is it has a higher fat content than many other diets. Food stays in the stomach for longer as fat and is digested slowly, thus provides a sense of fullness. On top of that, proteins promote the secretion cholecystokinin, which is a hormone that aids in regulating appetite. It is also believed that the ketogenic diet helps to suppress your appetite by continuous blunting of appetite. There is increased appetite in the initial stages of the diet, which decreases over time.

Changes in Cholesterol Levels

This is kind of on the fence between good and bad. This is because the ketogenic diet involves a high fat intake which makes people wonder about the effect on blood lipids and its potential to increase chances of heart disease and strokes, among others. Several major components play a lead role in determining this, which is: LDL, HDL, and blood triglyceride levels. Heart disease correlates with high levels of LDL and cholesterol. On the other hand, high levels of HDL are seen as protection from diseases caused by cholesterol levels. The impacts of the diet on cholesterol are not properly known. Some research has shown that there is no change in cholesterol levels while others have said that there is change. If you stay in deep ketosis for a very long period of time, your blood lipids will increase, but you will have to go through some negative effects of the ketogenic diet which will be corrected when the diet is over. If a person does not remain following the diet strictly for like ten years, he/she will not experience any cholesterol problems. It is difficult to differentiate the difference between diet and weight loss in general. The effect of the ketogenic diet on cholesterol has been boiled down to if you lose fat on the ketogenic diet then your cholesterol levels will go down, and if you don't lose fat, then your cholesterol levels will go up. Strangely, women have a larger cholesterol level addition than men, while both are on a diet. As there is no absolute conclusion on the effect of the ketogenic diet on cholesterol, you are advised to have your blood lipid levels constantly checked for any bad effects. Blood lipid levels should be checked before starting the diet and about eight weeks after starting. If repeated results show a worsening of lipid levels, then you should abandon the diet or substitute saturated fats with unsaturated fats.

Increase Body Energy Level

We compared briefly the difference between the glucose molecules synthesized from a high carbohydrates intake versus ketones produced on the Keto diet. Ketones are made by the liver and use fat molecules you already have stored. This makes them much more energy-rich and a lasting source of fuel compared to glucose, a simple sugar molecule. These ketones can give you a burst of energy physically as well as mentally allow you to have greater focus, clarity, and attention to detail.

Boost Brain Function and Mental Clarity

Like we elaborated earlier, the energy-rich ketones can boost the body's physical and mental levels of alertness. Research has shown that Keto is a much better energy source for the brain than simple sugar glucose molecules are. With nearly 75% of your diet coming from healthy fats, the brain's neural cells and mitochondria have a better source of energy to be able to function at the highest level. Some studies have tested patients on the Keto diet and found they had higher cognitive functioning, better memory recall, and were less susceptible to memory loss. The Keto diet can even decrease the occurrence of migraines which can be very detrimental to patients.

Slowing Down Aging Process

It almost sounds too good to be true, doesn't it? As you follow the ketogenic diet, it has been found that a low carb diet can lower the oxidative stress in the body. As this happens, it can increase one's lifespan. Studies show that as the insulin levels in the body lower, oxidative stress also lowers.

Reduce Inflammation

Inflammation on its own is a natural response by the body's immune system, but when it becomes uncontrollable, it can lead to an array of health problems, some severe, some minor. The many health concerns include acne, autoimmune conditions, arthritis, psoriasis, irritable bowel syndrome, and even acne and eczema. Often, removing sugars and carbohydrates from your diet can help patients of these diseases avoid flare-ups—and the good news is Keto does just that! A 2008 research study found that Keto decreased a blood marker linked to high inflammation in the body by nearly 40%. This is great news for people who may suffer from an inflammatory disease and are willing to change their diet to hopefully see improvement.

CHAPTER 4:

Practical Tips for Success

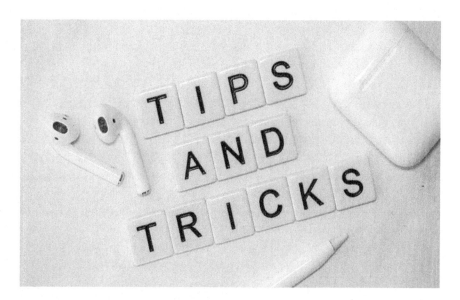

Nobody told you that life was going to be this way! But don't worry. There's still plenty of time to make amendments and take care of your health. Here are a couple of tips that will allow you to lead a healthier life in your fifties:

Start Building on Immunity

Every day, our body is exposed to free radicals and toxins from the environment. The added stress of work and family problems doesn't make it any easier for us. To combat this, it's essential that you start consuming healthy veggies that contain plenty of antioxidants and build a healthier immune system.

This helps ward off unwanted illnesses and diseases, allowing you to maintain good health.

Adding more healthy veggies to your keto diet will help you obtain a variety of minerals, vitamins and antioxidants.

Consider Quitting Smoking

It's never too late to try to quit smoking even if you are in your fifties. Once a smoker begins to quit, the body quickly starts to heal the previous damages caused by smoking.

Once you start quitting, you'll notice how you'll be able to breathe easier, while acquiring a better sense of smell and taste. Over the period of time, eliminating the habit of smoking can greatly reduce the risks of a high blood pressure, strokes and heart attack. Please note how these diseases are much more common among folks who are in the fifties and above when compared to younger folks.

Not to mention, quitting smoking will help you stay more active and enjoy better health with your friends and family.

Stay Social

We've already mentioned this before, but it's worth pondering on again and again. Aging can be a daunting process, and trying to get through it all on your own isn't particularly helpful. We urge you to stay in touch with friends and family or become a part of a local community club or network. Some older folks find it comforting to get an emotional support animal.

Being surrounded by people you love will give you a sense of belonging and will improve your mood. It'll also keep your mind and memory sharp as you engage in different conversations.

Health Screenings You Should Get After Your Fifties

Your fifties are considered the prime years of your life. Don't let the joy of these years be robbed away from you because of poor health. Getting simple tests done can go a long way in identifying any potential health problems that you may have. Here is a list of health screenings you should get done:

Check Your Blood Pressure

Your blood pressure is a reliable indicator of your heart health. In simple words, blood pressure is a measure of how fast blood travels through the artery walls. Very high or even very low blood pressure can be a sign of an underlying problem. Once you hit your 40s, you should have your blood pressure checked more often.

EKG

The EKG reveals your heart health and activity. Short for electrocardiogram, the EKG helps identify problems in the heart. The process works by highlighting any rhythm problems that may be in the heart such as poor heart muscles, improper blood flow or any other form of abnormality. Getting an EKG is also a predictive measure for understanding the chances of a heart attack. Since people starting their fifties are at greater risk of getting a heart attack, you should get yourself checked more often.

Mammogram

Mammograms help rule out the risks of breast cancer. Women who enter their fifties should ideally get a mammogram after every ten years. However, if you have a family history, it is advisable that you get one much earlier to rule out the possibilities of cancer.

Blood Sugar Levels

If you're somebody who used to grab a fast food meal every once in a while before you switched to keto, then you should definitely check your blood sugar levels more carefully. Blood sugar levels indicate whether or not you have diabetes. And you know how the saying goes, prevention is better than cure. It's best to clear these possibilities out of the way sooner than later.

Check for Osteoporosis

Unfortunately, as you grow older, you also become susceptible to a number of bone diseases. Osteoporosis is a bone-related condition in which bones begin to lose mass, becoming frail and weak. Owing to this, seniors become more prone to fractures. This can make even the smallest of falls detrimental to your health.

Annual Physical Exam

Your insurance must be providing coverage for your annual physical exam. So, there's no reason you should not take advantage of it. This checkup helps identify the state of your health. You'll probably be surprised by how much doctors can tell from a single blood test.

Prostate Screening Exam

Once men hit their fifties, they should be screened for prostate cancer (similar to how women should get a mammogram and pap smear). Getting a screening done becomes especially important if cancer runs in your family.

Eye Exam

As you start to age, you'll notice how your eyesight will start to deteriorate. It's quite likely that vision is not as sharp as it used to be. Ideally, you should have gotten your first eye exam during your 40s, but it isn't too late. Get one as soon as possible to prevent symptoms from escalating.

Be Wary of Any Weird Moles

While skin cancer can become a problem at any age, older adults should pay closer attention to any moles or unusual skin tags in their body. While most cancers can be easily treated, melanoma can be particularly quite dangerous.

If you have noticed any recent moles in your body that have changed in color, size or shape, make sure to visit the dermatologist.

Check Your Cholesterol Levels

Now, we've talked about this plenty of times, but it's worth mentioning again. High cholesterol levels can be dangerous to your health and can be an indicator for a number of diseases, things become more complicated for conditions that don't show particular symptoms. Just to be on the safe side, your total cholesterol levels should be below 200 mg per deciliter. Your doctor will take a simple blood test and will give you a couple of guidelines with the results. In case there is something to be worried about, you should make serious dietary and lifestyle changes in your life.

CHAPTER 5:

How Does Keto Diet Works?

We will focus on how this diet works and how your body transitions from one way of functioning to another.

As mentioned before, the ketogenic diet was used mainly to lower the incidence of seizures in epileptic children.

People wanted to check out how the keto diet would work w/ an entirely healthy person as things usually go.

This diet makes the body burn fats much faster than it does carbohydrates. The carbohydrates that we take in through food are turned into glucose, one of the leading "brain foods." So, once you start following the keto diet, food w/ reduced carbohydrates are forcing the liver to turn all the fats into fatty acids and ketone bodies. The ketones go to the brain and take the place of glucose, becoming the primary energy source.

This diet's primary purpose is to make your body switch from the way it used to function to an entirely new way of creating energy, keeping you healthy and alive.

Once you start following the ketogenic diet, you will notice that things are changing, first and foremost, in your mind. Before, carbohydrates were your main body 'fuel' and were used to create glucose so that your brain could function. Now you no longer feed yourself w/ them.

In the beginning, most people feel odd because their natural food is off the table. When your menu consists of more fats and proteins, it is natural to feel that something is missing.

Your brain alarms you that you haven't eaten enough and sends you signals that you are hungry. It is literally "panicking" and telling you that you are starving, which is not correct. You get to eat, and you get to eat plenty of good food, but not carbs.

This condition usually arises during the first day or two. Afterward, people get used to their new eating habits.

Once the brain "realizes" that carbs are no longer an option, it will focus on "finding" another abundant energy source: in this case, fats.

Not only is your food rich in fats, but your body contains stored fats in large amounts. As you consume more fats and fewer carbs, your body "runs" on the fats, both consumed and stored. The best thing is that, as the fats are used for energy, they are burned. This is how you get a double gain from this diet.

Usually, it will take a few days of consuming low-carb meals before you start seeing visible weight loss results. You will not even have to check your weight because the fat layers will be visibly reduced.

This diet requires you to lower your daily consumption of carbs to only 20 grams. For most people, this transition from a regular carb-rich diet can be quite a challenge. Most people are used to eating bread, pasta, rice, dairy products, sweets, soda, alcohol, and fruits, so quitting all these foods might be challenging.

However, this is all in your head. If you manage to win the "battle" w/ your mind and endure the diet for a few days, you will see that you no longer have cravings as time goes by. Plus, the weight loss and the fat burn will be a great motivation to continue w/ this diet.

The keto diet practically makes the body burn fats much faster than carbohydrates; the foods you consume w/ this diet are quite rich in fats. Carbs will be there, too, but at far lower levels than before. Foods rich in carbohydrates are the body's primary fuel or the brain's food. (Our bodies turn carbs into glucose.) Because there are hardly any carbohydrates in this diet, the body will have to find a substitute source of energy to keep itself alive. Many people who don't truly need to lose weight and are completely healthy still choose to follow the keto diet because it is a great way to keep their meals balanced. Also, it is the perfect way to cleanse the body of toxins, processed foods, sugars, and unnecessary carbs. The combination of these things is usually the main reason for heart failure, some cancers, diabetes, cholesterol, or obesity.

If you ask a nutritionist about this diet, they will recommend it without a doubt. So, if you feel like cleansing your body and starting a diet that will keep you healthy, well-fed, and slender, perhaps the keto diet should be your primary choice. And what is the best thing about it (besides the fact that you will balance your weight & lower the risk of many diseases)?

There is no yo-yo effect. The keto diet can be followed forever and has no side effects. It does not restrict you from following it for a few weeks or a month. Once you get your body to keto foods, you will not think about going back to the old ways of eating your meals.

Signs that You Are in Ketosis

Since the human body heavily depends on Carbs, it always takes time for the body to adapt according to the new ketogenic lifestyle. It's like changing the fuel of a machine when the body is switched to the ketogenic diet; it shows some different signs than usual, which are as follows:

Increased Urination

Ketones are normally known as a diuretic, which means that they help in the removal of the extra water out of the body through increased urination. So high levels of ketones mean more urination than normal. Due to ketosis, more acetoacetate is released about three times faster than the usual, which is excreted along w/ urine, and its release then causes more urination.

Dry Mouth

It is obvious that more urination means the loss of high amounts of water, which causes dehydration as more water is released out of the body due to ketosis. Along w/ those fluids, many metabolites and electrolytes are also excreted out of the body. Therefore, it is always recommended to increase the water consumption on a ketogenic diet, along w/ a good intake of electrolytes, to maintain the water levels of the body. It helps to incorporate more salty things (like pickles) into the meal.

Bad Breath

A ketone, which is known as acetone, is released through our breath. This ketone has a distinct smell, and it takes some time to go away. Due to ketosis, a high number of acetones are released through the breath, which causes bad breath. It can be reduced w/ the help of a fresh mouth.

Reduced Appetite and Lasting Energy

It is the clearest sign of ketosis. Since Fat molecules are high-energy macronutrients, each molecule is broken down to produce three times more energy than a carb molecule. Therefore, a person feels more energized round the clock.

CHAPTER 6:

Common Mistakes

As you are well aware of at this point, there are some incredible benefits that come with the Ketogenic Diet. When you first start this diet, you are going to make a number of different mistakes. Whether you eat too many carbs, fall out of ketosis, or even just ditch your entire diet for the day, that is okay! What isn't okay is giving up this diet for good. Luckily because you are here, you will now learn some of the common mistakes people make on the Ketogenic Diet and how to avoid them in the first place!

Excess Protein

Excess protein intake is probably one of the biggest mistakes individuals make on this diet, especially when they are first getting started on the Ketogenic Diet. This is due to the fact that individuals give too much credit to the process of gluconeogenesis. You may be asking yourself, gluco-what? The method of gluconeogenesis is the process where your liver converts the protein you consume into blood glucose.

The key here is to realize that gluconeogenesis will only operate when it is on-demand, not when it is available. Essentially, this means that just because you ate a lot of protein in one day does not mean that it will automatically be converted into glucose. This process will only occur if your body needs glucose in the first place. So, while protein is going to be necessary on your diet, it should be consumed in moderation.

Excess Nuts and Dairy

As you learned earlier, dairy and nuts are both going to be significant sources of fats, but with that in mind, remember that these two foods are both calorie-dense. For this reason, it can become incredibly easy to overindulge on these foods, causing weight gain. Much like with protein, you can still enjoy these foods, but in moderation. If you feel dairy and nuts are trigger foods for you, you may want to try avoiding them for the first few weeks that you are following a Ketogenic Diet.

Adaption Time

While starting any diet, it is important not to expect results overnight. As you begin the Ketogenic Diet, you are going to be putting your body through some pretty profound changes. With such a significant difference, may come considerable struggles. Luckily, our bodies are pretty hardy when it comes to dealing with change and adapting to a different diet. It may seem frustrating at first, but you need to give your body time to adjust to your new diet. Remember that you are not just changing your diet; you are changing your overall fuel source! Give yourself some time, and the benefits will come before you know it.

Excess Carbohydrates

At this point, you are well aware that the Ketogenic Diet is based around limiting carbs. Unfortunately, this can be very tricky when you are first starting out. As you learn what you can and cannot eat, you can expect to be in and out of ketosis fairly often. While this may be frustrating, you may want to take a closer look at your diet.

The key here is figuring out the maximum net carbs you can have in a day, depending on your activity level and metabolism. In the chapter to follow, we will be going more into depth on this subject. For general purposes, you will want to stay below 20 net carbs in a day to help you stay in ketosis. Once you become adapted to your new diet, you will learn precisely what your personal limit is and will excel from that point.

Snacking

In general, it is a pretty common habit to snack throughout the day. For some, this is to cure anxiety, and for others, its due to pure boredom! Snacking is also included in a number of different leisure activities, from dining out with friends to simply watching a movie.

If you are looking to lose weight on the Ketogenic Diet, you may want to limit your snacking. No matter what diet you follow, weight loss is equal to burning more calories than you consume. This rule is no different on your new diet.

Dehydration and Electrolytes

In the third chapter of this book, we will be tackling the dreaded Keto Flu. When you are first starting out, you will want to make sure you are staying hydrated and getting in enough electrolytes. The ketogenic diet has a dietetic effect, and when you lose water, you lose electrolytes. The three electrolytes you will want to focus on include magnesium, potassium, and sodium. Some of the best sources of potassium will be salmon, broccoli, spinach, and avocado. As long as you keep water and electrolytes consumption up, it will help you drastically while dealing with the symptoms of the Keto Flu.

Mindset

Finally, the most prominent mistake people make it not having the right mindset. If you are negative and miserable about your new diet, there is no way that you are going to stick with it! Instead, try your best to have a winner's mindset. This meaning that you start the diet off with clear goals and a reason behind your why. As you begin, ask yourself what is motivating you to begin this diet in the first place. What is going to drive you? Who are you doing this for? When you want to succeed at this diet more than anything else in the world, that is where you will find your success.

Now that you have a thorough understanding of Ketogenic Basics, it is time to learn how the Ketogenic Diet can help those of us who are over the age of 50! Yes, we are getting older, but life isn't over yet! There are still plenty of reasons to boost our health and perhaps live even better than when we were younger. If that sounds good to you, let's dive right into the next chapter.

CHAPTER 7:

Recommended Keto Foods

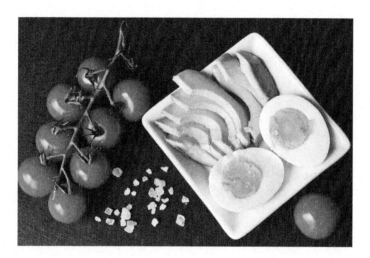

To make the most of your diet, there are prohibited foods, and others that are allowed, but in limited quantities. Here are the foods allowed in the ketogenic diet:

Food Allowed in Unlimited Quantities

Lean or Fatty Meats

No matter which meat you choose, it contains no carbohydrates so that you can have fun! Pay attention to the quality of your meat, and the amount of fat. Alternate between fatty meats and lean meats!

Here are some examples of lean meats:

- Beef: sirloin steak, roast beef, 5% minced steak, roast, flank steak, tenderloin, grisons meat, tripe, kidneys
- Horse: roti, steak
- Pork: tenderloin, bacon, kidneys
- Veal: cutlet, shank, tenderloin, sweetbread, liver
- Chicken and turkey: cutlet, skinless thigh, ham
- Rabbit

Here are some examples of fatty meats:
- Lamb: leg, ribs, brain
- Beef: minced steak 10, 15, 20%, ribs, rib steak, tongue, marrow
- Pork: ribs, brain, dry ham, black pudding, white pudding, bacon, terrine, rillettes, salami, sausage, sausages, and merguez
- Veal: roast, paupiette, marrow, brain, tongue, dumplings
- Chicken and turkey: thigh w/ skin
- Guinea fowl
- Capon
- Turkey
- Goose: foie gras

Lean or Fatty Fish

The fish does not contain carbohydrates so that you can consume unlimited! As w/ meat, there are lean fish and fatty fish, pay attention to the amount of fat you eat and remember to vary your intake of fish. Oily fish have the advantage of containing a lot of good cholesterol, so it is beneficial for protection against cardiovascular disease! It will be advisable to consume fatty fish more than lean fish, to be able to manage your protein intake: if you consume lean fish, you will have a significant protein intake and little lipids, whereas w/ fatty fish, you will have a balanced protein and fat intake!

Here are some examples of lean fish:
- Cod
- Colin
- Sea bream
- Whiting
- Sole
- Turbot
- Limor career
- Location
- Pike
- Ray

Here are some examples of oily fish:
- Swordfish
- Salmon
- Tuna
- Trout
- Monkfish
- Herring
- Mackerel
- Cod
- Sardine

Eggs

The eggs contain no carbohydrates, so you can consume as much as you want. It is often said that eggs are full of cholesterol and that you have to limit their intake, but the more cholesterol you eat, the less your body will produce by itself! In addition, it's not just poor-quality cholesterol so that you can consume 6 per week without risk! And if you want to eat more but you are afraid of your cholesterol, and I have not convinced you, remove the yellow!

Vegetables and Raw Vegetables

Yes, you can eat vegetables. But you have to be careful which ones: you can eat leafy vegetables (salad, spinach, kale, red cabbage, Chinese cabbage...) and flower vegetables (cauliflower, broccoli, Romanesco cabbage...) as well as avocado, cucumbers, zucchini or leeks, which do not contain many carbohydrates.

The Oils

It's oil, so it's only fat, so it's unlimited to eat, but choose your oil wisely! I prefer olive oil, rapeseed, nuts, sunflower or sesame, for example!

Foods Authorized in Moderate Quantities

The Cold Cuts

As you know, there is bad cholesterol in cold meats, so you will need to moderate your intake: eat it occasionally!

Fresh Cheeses and Plain Yogurts

Consume w/ moderation because they contain carbohydrates.

Nuts and Oilseeds

They have low levels of carbohydrates, but are rich in saturated fatty acids, that's why they should moderate their consumption. Choose almonds, hazelnuts, Brazil nuts or pecans.

Coconut (in Oil, Cream or Milk)

It contains saturated fatty acids, that's why we limit its consumption. Cream and coconut oil contain a lot of medium chain triglycerides (MCTs), which increase the level of ketones, essential to stay in ketosis.

Berries and Red Fruits

They contain carbohydrates, in reasonable quantities, but you should not abuse them to avoid ketosis (blueberries, blackberries, raspberries...).

CHAPTER 8:

Food and Beverage to Avoid

B ecause the diet is a keto, that means you need to avoid high-carbs food. Some of the food you avoid is even healthy, but it just contains too many carbs. Here is a list of typical food you should limit or avoid altogether.

Bread and Grains

No matter what form bread takes, they still pack a lot of carbs. The same applies to whole-grain as well because they are made from refined flour. So, if you want to eat bread, it is best to make keto variants at home instead. Grains such as rice, wheat, and oats pack a lot of carbs as well. So, limit or avoid that as well.

Fruits

Fruits are healthy for you. The problem is that some of those foods pack quite a lot of carbs such as banana, raisins, dates, mango, and pear. As a general rule, avoid sweet and dried fruits.

Vegetables

Vegetables are just as healthy for your body. For one, they make you feel full for longer, so they help suppress your appetite. But that also means you need to avoid or limit vegetables that are high in starch because they have more carbs than fiber. That includes corn, potato, sweet potato, and beets.

Pasta

As with any other convenient food, pasta is rich in carbs. So, spaghetti or any different types of pasta are not recommended when you are on your keto diet.

Cereal

Cereal is also a considerable offender because sugary breakfast cereals pack a lot of carbs. That also applies to "healthy cereals." Just because they use other words to describe their product does not mean that you should believe them. That also applies to oatmeal, whole-grain cereals, etc.

Beer

In reality, you can drink most alcoholic beverages in moderation without fear. Beer is an exception to this rule because it packs a lot of carbs. Carbs in beers or other liquid are considered liquid carbs, and they are even more dangerous than substantial carbs.

Sweetened Yogurt

Yogurt is very healthy because it is tasty and does not have that many carbs. The problem comes when you consume yogurt variants rich in carbs such as fruit-flavored, low-fat, sweetened, or nonfat yogurt. A single serving of sweetened yogurt contains as many carbs as a single serving of dessert.

Juice

Fruit juices are perhaps the worst beverage you can put into your system when you are on a keto diet. Another problem is that the brain does not process liquid carbs the same way as stable carbs. Substantial carbs can help suppress appetite, but liquid carbs will only put your need into overdrive.

Low-Fat and Fat-Free Salad Dressings

If you have to buy salads, keep in mind that commercial sauces pack more carbs than you think, especially the fat-free and low-fat variants.

Beans and Legumes

These are also very nutritious as they are rich in fiber. However, they are also rich in carbs. You may enjoy a small amount of them when you are on your keto diet, but don't exceed your carb limit.

Sugar

We mean sugar in any form, including honey. Foods that contain lots of sugar, such as cookies, candies, and cake, are forbidden on a keto diet or any other form of diet that is designed to lose weight. When you are on a keto diet, you need to keep in mind that your diet consists of food that is rich in fiber and nutritious. So, sugar is out of the question.

Chips and Crackers

These two are some of the most popular snacks. Some people did not realize that one packet of chips contains several servings and should not be all eaten in one go. The carbs can add up very quickly if you do not watch what you eat.

Milk

Milk also contains a lot of carbs on its own. Therefore, avoid it if you can even though milk is a good source of many nutrients such as calcium, potassium, and other B vitamins.

Gluten-Free Baked Goods

Gluten-free diets are trendy nowadays, but what many people don't seem to realize is that they pack quite a lot of carbs. That includes gluten-free bread, muffins, and other baked products. In reality, they contain even more carbs than their glutenous variant.

CHAPTER 9:

More About Keto Diet

Hormone Balance

With a more thorough understanding of how the ketogenic diet can help balance your hormones, it is time to learn how! By embracing the ketogenic life and applying these lessons to your everyday life, you will enjoy this diet in no time. Remember that while it will take some extra effort at first, it will be thoroughly worth it. The first thing you will want to do is focus on your diet! One of the most beneficial steps you can take is starting eating foods rich in probiotics. By doing this, you will keep your gut bacteria in check. Also, plan to eat more protein for about three days before your period, to help keep your hormones in check.

Another way you can help your hormone balance is to eat foods rich in calcium. Foods such as almonds, salmon, celery, sesame, and poppy can help with symptoms that are associated with mood swings. If you ever have questions, you can always test your hormone levels to make sure they are in check. The ones you will want to pay special attention to include cortisol, progesterone, estrogen, and SBHG. While this isn't diet-related, managing your stress levels is a vital part of balancing your hormones. Remember that stress had a major effect on your hormones, so you need to address the issue at hand. To help combat stress, remember to move your body, sleep well, and spend time with your loved ones.

Finally, you will want to test your pH levels. As we age, maintaining the alkalinity within your diet will be key. Alkalinity has a direct effect on your vitamin absorption, lowers inflammation, improved bone density, and helps you maintain a healthy weight. Luckily on the ketogenic diet, you will balance this in your diet.

Menopause

There's a lot that the ketogenic diet does to help you reach a healthy and balanced weight and stay there: restore insulin levels of sensitivity, build and maintain muscle mass and lower inflammation. A woman who consumes way too many carbohydrates can jump-start menopause signs. Let's have a look at how a ketogenic diet can aid with the signs and symptoms of this menopause.

Way # 1 – Controlling Insulin Levels

By going on a ketogenic diet, women with PCOS (Polycistic Ovarie Syndrome) can help regulate their hormones. Research studied the effect of low-glycemic diets has shown this impact. PCOS triggers insulin sensitivity concerns, to be helped by insulin-reducing properties of low-glycemic carbohydrates.

Way # 2 – You'll Have More Energy

Our bodies will experience widely known energy dips if we fuel them with mainly sugar and carbohydrates. Especially if you take in quick and refined sugars (think about carrot cake, cupcakes, crackers, bread, candy, etc.). Changes in blood glucose can stop by receiving a steady amount of sugar. High blood glucose makes the body send insulin to the pancreas, which then takes care of how muscular tissue and fat cells absorb sugar.

The reaction to the consumption of carbs is a powerful release of insulin to make sure that the body can properly manage the transport of the extra sugar. With blood sugar levels down, the body will signal that it requires more sugar. This means you'll experience many energy lows and highs in one day. This produces a reduced energy level.

Way # 3 – Fat Burning

Menopause can trigger the metabolic process to change and reduce. One of the most common complaints of the menopause is an increase in body weight and abdominal fat. A lower level of estrogen typically causes weight gain. A diet with little or no carbohydrates is very efficient for decreasing body fat. Ketosis reduces appetite by controlling the production of the 'cravings hormonal agent' called ghrelin. You are less hungry while in ketosis.

Way # 4 – Reduction in Hot Flashes

Nobody totally understands hot flashes and why they take place. Hormonal changes that impact the hypothalamus; most likely have something to do with this. The hypothalamus manages the body's temperature level. Changes in hormonal agents can also disrupt this thermostat. This ends up being more sensitive to modifications in body temperature levels.

Ketone, in which its production stimulates throughout a ketogenic diet, creates a very potent source of energy for the mind. Scientists have shown that ketones act to help the hypothalamus. The body can manage its own temperature level better. The presence of ketones works to make your body's thermostat better.

Way # 5 – Excellent Night's Rest

Thanks to a much steadier blood sugar level, you will improve rest while on a ketogenic diet. With even more balanced hormones and much less warm flashes, you will sleep better. Reduced stress and an enhanced well-being are 2 of the benefits of better sleep.

Autophagy

Autophagy or auto phagocytosis is one of the essential processes in the human body to keep the cells healthy and efficient. It is a kind of "self-digestion program" that cleanses and detoxifies the cells. In the single-cell, autophagy causes removal and modification, as well as the provision of amino acids. This happens with temporary containment of the food supply, as is the case during fasting, as well as with the number of certain foods. Autophagy is performed in any cell, and factors such as stress, periods of growth, or pregnancy also affect and enhance the intensity of this process.

Without autophagy, metabolic diseases, cancers, or even diabetes would be more common as the human body would not be able to dispose of its "cell wastes" in this case. Autophagy thereby assumes a protective cell-cleaning function.

CHAPTER 10:

Breakfast

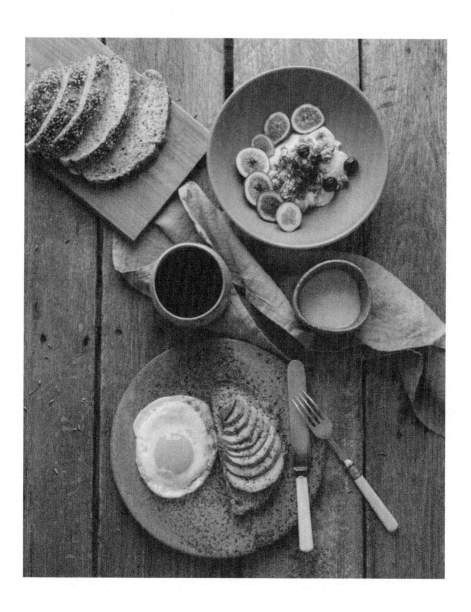

1. Breakfast Omelette with Mushrooms

Preparation Time: 10 minutes
Cooking Time: 20 minutes
Servings: 1
Ingredients:
- 3 eggs, whisked
- 1 oz. butter, for frying
- 1 oz. cheese, shredded
- 2 Tbsp. yellow onion, chopped
- 5 small (4 big) mushrooms, sliced
- Salt and black pepper, to taste

Directions:
1. In a separate bowl, crack the eggs. Then add salt and pepper and whisk the mixture until frothy.
2. Melt the butter in a pan on medium heat.
3. Add the onion and mushrooms. Stir and cook for 5 minutes until the onion is translucent and the mushrooms are soft.
4. Pour the egg mixture into the pan and cover with shredded cheese when the eggs are starting to become firm.
5. Fry until the eggs are almost firm.
6. Fold the omelette in half and remove from the heat.

Nutrition:
- Carbohydrates: 4g
- Fat: 43g
- Protein: 25g
- Calories: 510

2. Morning Coconut Porridge

Preparation Time: 1 minute
Cooking Time: 5 minutes
Servings: 1
Ingredients:

- 1 egg, beaten
- 1 Tbsp. coconut milk
- 2 Tbsp. coconut flour
- 2 tsp butter
- 1 cup water
- 1 pinch salt
- 2 Tbsp. flax seeds
- Blueberries and raspberries

Directions:

1. Put the flax seeds, coconut flour, water, and salt into a saucepan.
2. Heat this mixture until it has thickened slightly
3. Remove the mixture from the heat. Add beaten egg and put it on the stove again. Whisk slowly until you get a creamy texture.
4. Remove from the heat, add the butter and stir.
5. Serve with coconut milk, blueberries, and raspberries.

Nutrition:

- Carbohydrates: 6g
- Fat: 27g
- Protein: 15g
- Calories: 486

3. Dairy-Free Pizza

Preparation Time: 10 minutes
Cooking Time: 15 minutes
Servings: 2
Ingredients:

- 4 eggs
- 2 cups cauliflower, grated
- 2 Tbsp. coconut flour
- 1 Tbsp. psyllium husk powder
- 2 pinches salt
- Smoked salmon
- Avocado
- Spinach
- Herbs

Directions:

1. Heat the oven to 350°F and line the pizza tray with parchment.
2. Take a mixing bowl and place the eggs, cauliflower, coconut flour, and psyllium husk powder into it. Mix all the ingredients, add salt, and leave for 5 minutes until the mixture thickens up.
3. Pour your base for the breakfast pizza onto the tray.
4. Bake your pizza for 15 minutes.
5. Remove it and decorate with smoked salmon, avocado, spinach, and herbs.

Nutrition:

- Carbohydrates: 7g
- Fat: 55g
- Protein: 15g
- Calories: 226

4. Sesame Keto Bagels

Preparation Time: 10 minutes
Cooking Time: 15 minutes
Servings: 6
Ingredients:
- 2 cups almond flour
- 3 eggs
- 1 Tbsp. baking powder
- 2½ cups Mozzarella cheese, shredded
- ½ cream cheese, cubed
- 1 pinch salt
- 2-3 tsp sesame seeds

Directions:
1. Preheat the oven to 425°F.
2. Use a medium bowl to whisk the almond flour and baking powder. Add the mozzarella cheese and cubed cream cheese into a large bowl, mix and microwave for 90 seconds. Place 2 eggs into the almond mixture and stir it thoroughly to form a dough.
3. Part your dough into 6 portions and make into balls. Press every dough ball slightly to make a hole in the center and put your ball on the baking mat.
4. Brush the top of every bagel with the remaining egg and top with sesame seeds.
5. Bake for about 15 minutes.

Nutrition:
- Carbohydrates: 9g
- Fat: 39g
- Protein: 23g
- Calories: 469

5. Baked Eggs in Avocado Halves

Preparation Time: 10 minutes
Cooking Time: 15 minutes
Servings: 2
Ingredients:

- 1 large avocado
- 2 eggs
- 3 oz. bacon
- 1 small tomato, chopped
- 1 pinch salt and paper
- ½ oz. lettuce, shredded

Directions:

1. Fry the bacon and cut it. Put aside.
2. Warm your oven to 375°F.
3. Cut the avocado in two halves and make a large hole in each half to place the egg in it.
4. Put avocado halves onto a baking sheet, place eggs, add salt and pepper. Cover the eggs with chopped tomatoes and bacon.
5. Bake for 15 minutes and top your avocadoes with shredded lettuce at the end.

Nutrition:

- Carbohydrates: 7g
- Fat: 72g
- Protein: 26g
- Calories: 810

6. Spicy Cream Cheese Pancakes

Preparation Time: 15 minutes
Cooking Time: 20 minutes
Servings: 2
Ingredients:

- 3 eggs
- 9 Tbsp. cottage cheese
- Salt, to taste
- ½ Tbsp. psyllium husk powder
- Butter, for frying
- 4 oz. cream cheese
- 1 Tbsp. green pesto
- 1 Tbsp. olive oil
- ¼ red onion, finely sliced
- Black pepper, to taste

Directions:

1. Combine cream cheese, olive oil, and pesto. Put this mixture aside.
2. Blend eggs, psyllium husk powder, cottage cheese, and salt until the mixture is smooth. Leave it for 5 minutes.
3. Heat the butter in the pan and put several dollops of cottage cheese batter into the pan. Fry for a few minutes each side.
4. Top your pancakes with a large amount of cream cheese mixture and several red onion slices.
5. Add black pepper and olive oil.

Nutrition:

- Carbohydrates: 7g
- Fat: 38g
- Protein: 18g
- Calories: 449

7. Bracing Ginger Smoothie

Preparation Time: 5 minutes
Cooking Time: 5 minutes.
Servings: 2
Ingredients:

- ⅓ Cup coconut cream
- ⅔ Cup water
- 2 Tbsp. lime juice
- 1 oz. spinach, frozen
- 2 Tbsp. ginger, grated

Directions:

1. Blend all the ingredients. Add 1 Tbsp. lime at first and increase the amount if necessary.
2. Top with grated ginger and enjoy your smoothie!

Nutrition:

- Carbohydrates: 3g Fat: 8g
- Protein: 1g Calories: 82

8. Morning Coffee with Cream

Preparation Time: 0 minutes
Cooking Time: 5 minutes
Servings: 1
Ingredients:

- ¾ cup coffee
- ¼ cup whipping cream

Directions:

1. Make your favorite coffee.
2. Pour the heavy cream in a small saucepan and heat slowly until you get a frothy texture.
3. Pour the hot cream in a big cup, add coffee and enjoy your morning drink.

Nutrition:

- Carbohydrates: 2g Fat: 21g
- Protein: 2g Calories: 202

9. Cheesy Breakfast Muffins

Preparation Time: 15 minutes
Cooking Time: 12 minutes
Servings: 6
Ingredients:

- 4 tablespoons melted butter
- 3/4 tablespoon baking powder
- 1 cup almond flour
- 2 large eggs, lightly beaten
- 2 ounces cream cheese mixed with 2 tablespoons heavy whipping cream
- A handful of shredded Mexican blend cheese

Directions:

1. Preheat the oven to 400°F. Grease 6 muffin tin cups with melted butter and set aside.
2. Combine the baking powder and almond flour in a bowl. Stir well and set aside.
3. Stir together four tablespoons melted butter, eggs, shredded cheese, and cream cheese in a separate bowl.
4. The egg and the dry mixture must be combined using a hand mixer to beat until it is creamy and well blended.
5. The mixture must be scooped into the greased muffin cups evenly.

Nutrition:

- Calories: 214
- Fat: 15.6g
- Fiber: 3.1g
- Carbohydrates: 5.1g
- Protein: 9.5g

10. Spinach, Mushroom, and Goat Cheese Frittata

Preparation Time: 15 minutes
Cooking Time: 20 minutes
Servings: 5
Ingredients:
- 2 tablespoons olive oil
- 1 cup fresh mushrooms, sliced
- 6 bacon slices, cooked and chopped
- 1 cup spinach, shredded
- 10 large eggs, beaten
- 1/2 cup goat cheese, crumbled
- Pepper and salt

Directions:
1. Preheat the oven to 350°F.
2. Heat oil and add the mushrooms and fry for 3 minutes until they start to brown, stirring frequently.
3. Fold in the bacon and spinach and cook for about 1 to 2 minutes, or until the spinach is wilted.
4. Slowly pour in the beaten eggs and cook for 3 to 4 minutes. Making use of a spatula, lift the edges for allowing uncooked egg to flow underneath.
5. Top with the goat cheese, then sprinkle the salt and pepper to season.
6. Bake in the preheated oven for about 15 minutes until lightly golden brown around the edges.

Nutrition:
- Calories: 265
- Fat: 11.6g
- Fiber: 8.6g
- Carbohydrates: 5.1g
- Protein: 12.9g

11. Cheesy Broccoli Muffins

Preparation Time: 15 minutes
Cooking Time: 20 minutes
Servings: 6
Ingredients:

- 2 tablespoons unsalted butter
- 6 large organic eggs
- 1/2 cup heavy whipping cream
- 1/2 cup Parmesan cheese, grated
- Salt and ground black pepper, as required
- 11/4 cups broccoli, chopped
- 2 tablespoons fresh parsley, chopped
- 1/2 cup Swiss cheese, grated

Directions:

1. Grease a 12-cup muffin tin.
2. In a bowl or container, put in the cream, eggs, Parmesan cheese, salt, and black pepper, and beat until well combined.
3. Divide the broccoli and parsley in the bottom of each prepared muffin cup evenly.
4. Top with the egg mixture, followed by the Swiss cheese.
5. Let the muffins bake for about 20 minutes, rotating the pan once halfway through.
6. Carefully, invert the muffins onto a serving platter and serve warm.

Nutrition:

- Calories: 241
- Fat: 11.5g
- Fiber: 8.5g
- Carbohydrates: 4.1g
- Protein: 11.1g

12. Berry Chocolate Breakfast Bowl

Preparation Time: 10 minutes
Cooking Time: 0 minutes
Servings: 2
Ingredients:
- 1/2 cup strawberries, fresh or frozen
- 1/2 cup blueberries, fresh or frozen
- 1 cup unsweetened almond milk
- Sugar-free maple syrup to taste
- 2 tbsp. unsweetened cocoa powder
- 1 tbsp. cashew nuts for topping

Directions:
1. The berries must be divided into four bowls, pour on the almond milk.
2. Drizzle with the maple syrup and sprinkle the cocoa powder on top, a tablespoon per bowl.
3. Top with the cashew nuts and enjoy immediately.

Nutrition:
- Calories: 287
- Fat: 5.9g
- Fiber: 11.4g
- Carbohydrates: 3.1g
- Protein: 4.2g

13. "Coco-Nut" Granola

Preparation Time: 10 minutes
Cooking Time: 60 minutes
Servings: 8
Ingredients:

- 2 cups shredded unsweetened coconut
- 1 cup sliced almonds
- 1 cup raw sunflower seeds
- 1/2 cup raw pumpkin seeds
- 1/2 cup walnuts
- 1/2 cup melted coconut oil
- 10 drops liquid stevia
- 1 teaspoon ground cinnamon
- 1/2 teaspoon ground nutmeg

Directions:

1. Preheat the oven to 250°F. Line 2 baking sheets with parchment paper. Set aside.
2. Toss all the ingredients together.
3. The granola will then put into baking sheets and spread it out evenly.
4. Bake the granola for about 1 hr.

Nutrition:

- Calories: 131
- Fat: 4.1g
- Fiber: 5.8g
- Carbohydrates: 2.8g
- Protein: 5.6g

CHAPTER 11:

Lunch

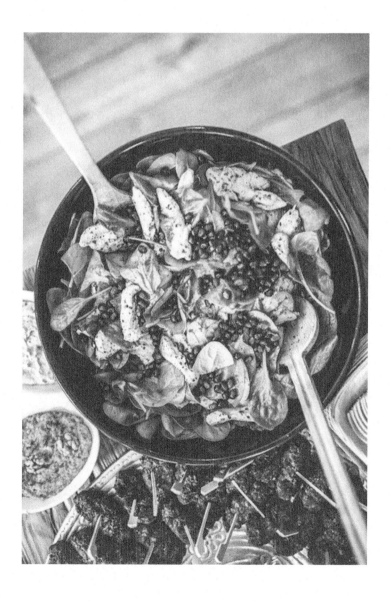

14. Cheesy Chicken Cauliflower

Preparation Time: 5 minutes
Cooking Time: 10 minutes
Servings: 4
Ingredients:
- 2 cups cauliflower florets, chopped
- ½ cup red bell pepper, chopped
- 1 cup roasted chicken, shredded
- ¼ cup shredded cheddar cheese
- 1 tablespoon. Butter
- 1 tablespoon. Sour cream
- Salt and pepper to taste

Directions:
1. Stir fry the cauliflower and peppers in the butter over medium heat until the veggies are tender.
2. Add the chicken and cook until the chicken is warmed through.
3. Add the remaining **Ingredients:** and stir until the cheese is melted.
4. Serve warm.

Nutrition:
- Calories: 144kcal
- Carbs: 4g
- Fat: 8.5g
- Protein: 13.2g

15. Chicken Soup

Preparation Time: 10 minutes
Cooking Time: 25 minutes
Servings: 6
Ingredients:

- 4 cups roasted chicken, shredded
- 2 tablespoons. Butter
- 2 celery stalks, chopped
- 1 cup mushrooms, sliced
- 4 cups green cabbage, cut into strips
- 2 garlic cloves, minced
- 6 cups chicken broth
- 1 carrot, sliced
- Salt and pepper to taste
- 1 tablespoon. Garlic powder
- 1 tablespoon. Onion powder

Directions:

1. Sauté the celery, mushrooms and garlic in the butter in a pot over medium heat for 4 minutes.
2. Add broth, carrots, garlic powder, onion powder, salt, and pepper.
3. Simmer for 10 minutes or until the vegetables are tender.
4. Add the chicken and cabbage and simmer for another 10 minutes or until the cabbage is tender.
5. Servings warm.
6. It can be refrigerated for up to 3 days or frozen for up to 1 month.

Nutrition:

- Calories: 279kcal
- Carbs: 7.5g
- Fat: 12.3g
- Protein: 33.4g

16. Chicken Avocado Salad

Preparation Time: 7 minutes
Cooking Time: 10 minutes
Servings: 4
Ingredients:
- 1 cup roasted chicken, shredded
- 1 bacon strip, cooked and chopped
- 1/2 medium avocado, chopped
- ¼ cup cheddar cheese, grated
- 1 hard-boiled egg, chopped
- 1 cup romaine lettuce, chopped
- 1 tablespoon. Olive oil
- 1 tablespoon. Apple cider vinegar
- Salt and pepper to taste

Directions:
1. Create the dressing by mixing apple cider vinegar, oil, salt and pepper.
2. Combine all the other ingredients in a mixing bowl.
3. Drizzle with the dressing and toss. Servings.
4. It can be refrigerated for up to 3 days.

Nutrition:
- Calories: 220kcal
- Carbs: 2.8g
- Fat: 16.7g
- Protein: 14.8g

17. Chicken Broccoli Dinner

Preparation Time: 10 minutes
Cooking Time: 5 minutes
Servings: 1
Ingredients:

- 1 roasted chicken leg
- ½ cup broccoli florets
- ½ tablespoon. Unsalted butter softened
- 2 garlic cloves, minced
- Salt and pepper to taste

Directions:

1. Boil the broccoli in lightly salted water for 5 minutes. Drain the water from the pot and keep the broccoli in the pool. Keep the lid on to keep the broccoli warm.
2. Mix all the butter, garlic, salt and pepper in a small bowl to create garlic butter.
3. Place the chicken, broccoli and garlic butter. Servings.

Nutrition:

- Calories: 257kcal
- Carbs: 5.1g
- Fat: 14g
- Protein: 27.4g

18. Lemon Baked Salmon

Preparation Time: 10 minutes
Cooking Time: 30 minutes
Servings: 4
Ingredients:

- 1 lb. salmon
- 1 tablespoon. Olive oil
- Salt and pepper to taste
- 1 tablespoon. Butter
- 1 lemon, thinly sliced
- 1 tablespoon. Lemon juice

Directions:

1. Preheat your oven to 400 degrees F.
2. Grease a baking dish with the olive oil and place the salmon skin-side down.
3. Season the salmon with salt and pepper then top with the lemon slices.
4. Slice half the butter and place over the salmon.
5. Bake for 20minutes or until the salmon flakes easily.
6. Melt the remaining butter in a saucepan. When it starts to bubble, remove from heat and allow to cool before adding the lemon juice.
7. Drizzle the lemon butter over the salmon and servings warm.

Nutrition:

- Calories: 211kcal
- Carbs: 1.5g
- Fat: 13.5g
- Protein: 22.2g

19. Cauliflower Mash

Preparation Time: 10 minutes
Cooking Time: 5 minutes
Servings: 8
Ingredients:

- 4 cups cauliflower florets, chopped
- 1 cup grated parmesan cheese
- 6 tablespoons. Butter
- ½ lemon, juice and zest
- Salt and pepper to taste

Directions:

1. Boil the cauliflower in lightly salted water over high heat for 5 minutes or until the florets are tender but still firm.
2. Strain the cauliflower in a colander and add the cauliflower to a food processor
3. Add the remaining ingredients and pulse the mixture to a smooth and creamy consistency
4. Servings with protein like salmon, chicken or meatballs.
5. It can be refrigerated for up to 3 days.

Nutrition:

- Calories: 101kcal
- Carbs: 3.1g
- Fat: 9.5g
- Protein: 2.2g

20. Baked Salmon

Preparation Time: 10 minutes
Cooking Time: 10 minutes
Servings: 4
Ingredients:

- Cooking spray
- 3 garlic cloves, minced
- ¼ cup butter
- 1 teaspoon lemon zest
- 2 tablespoons lemon juice
- 4 salmon fillets
- Salt and pepper to taste
- 2 tablespoons parsley, chopped

Directions:

1. Preheat your oven to 425 degrees F.
2. Grease the pan with cooking spray.
3. In a bowl, mix the garlic, butter, and lemon zest and lemon juice.
4. Sprinkle salt and pepper on salmon fillets.
5. Drizzle with the lemon butter sauce.
6. Bake in the oven for 12 minutes.
7. Garnish with parsley before serving.

Nutrition:

- Calories: 345
- Total Fat: 22.7g
- Saturated Fat: 8.9g
- Cholesterol: 109mg
- Sodium: 163mg
- Total Carbohydrate: 1.2g
- Dietary Fiber: 0.2g
- Total Sugars: 0.2g
- Protein: 34.9g
- Potassium: 718mg

21. Slow Cooker Chilli

Preparation Time: 15 minutes
Cooking Time: 6 hours and 15 minutes
Servings: 6 servings
Ingredients:

- 2 ½ lbs. ground beef
- 1 red onion, diced
- 5 garlic cloves, minced
- 1 ½ c celery, diced
- 1 6-ounce can tomato paste
- 1 14.5 oz. can diced tomatoes with green chilies
- 1 14.5 oz. can stewed tomatoes
- 4 T chili powder
- 2 T ground cumin
- 2 t salt
- 1 t garlic powder
- 1 t onion powder
- 3 t cayenne pepper
- 1 t red pepper flakes

Directions:

1. Cook ground beef in a large skillet.
2. Add onion, garlic, and celery and cook until ground beef browned
3. Drain the fat from the beef
4. Place beef and vegetable mixture into the slow cooker set on a low setting.
5. Add tomatoes and seasonings then stir to mix.
6. Place the lid on the slow cooker and cook on low for 6 hours.
7. Serve with cheese on top if desired. Adjust the red pepper to taste.

Nutrition:

- Calories: 137
- Carbohydrates: 4.7g
- Protein: 16g
- Fat: 5g

CHAPTER 12:

Dinner

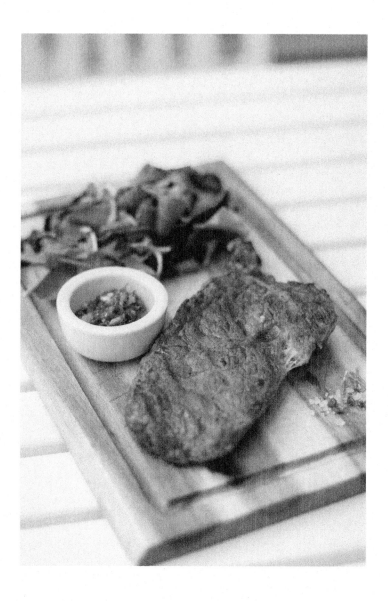

22. Beef-Stuffed Mushrooms

Preparation Time: 20 minutes
Cooking Time: 25 minutes
Servings: 4
Ingredients:

- 4 mushrooms, stemmed
- 3 tablespoons olive oil, divided
- 1 yellow onion, sliced thinly
- 1 red bell pepper, cut into strips
- 1 green bell pepper, cut into strips
- Salt and pepper to taste
- 8 oz. beef, sliced thinly
- 3 oz. provolone cheese, sliced
- Chopped parsley

Directions:

1. Preheat your oven to 350 degrees F.
2. Arrange the mushrooms on a baking pan.
3. Brush with oil.
4. Add the remaining oil to a pan over medium heat.
5. Cook onion and bell peppers for 5 minutes.
6. Season with salt and pepper.
7. Place onion mixture on a plate.
8. Cook the beef in the pan for 5 minutes.
9. Sprinkle with salt and pepper.
10. Add the onion mixture back to the pan.
11. Mix well.
12. Fill the mushrooms with the beef mixture and cheese.
13. Bake in the oven for 15 minutes.

Nutrition:

- Calories: 333 Total Fat: 20.3g
- Saturated Fat: 6.7g
- Cholesterol: 61mg
- Sodium: 378mg
- Total Carbohydrate: 8.2g
- Dietary Fiber: 3.7g
- Protein: 25.2g
- Total Sugars: 7g
- Potassium: 789mg

23. Rib Roast

Preparation Time: 15 minutes
Cooking Time: 3 hours
Servings: 8
Ingredients:
- 1 rib roast
- Salt to taste
- 12 garlic cloves, chopped
- 2 teaspoons lemon zest
- 6 tablespoons fresh rosemary, chopped
- 5 sprigs thyme

Directions:
1. Preheat your oven to 325 degrees F.
2. Season all sides of the rib roast with salt.
3. Place the rib roast in a baking pan.
4. Sprinkle with garlic, lemon zest and rosemary.
5. Add herb sprigs on top.
6. Roast for 3 hours.
7. Let rest for a few minutes and then slice and serve.

Nutrition:
- Calories: 329
- Total Fat: 27g
- Saturated Fat: 9g
- Cholesterol: 59mg
- Sodium: 498mg
- Total Carbohydrate: 5.3g
- Dietary Fiber: 1.8g
- Protein: 18g
- Total Sugars: 2g
- Potassium: 493mg

24. Beef Stir Fry

Preparation Time: 15 minutes
Cooking Time: 10 minutes
Servings: 4
Ingredients:

- 1 tablespoon soy sauce
- 1 tablespoon ginger, minced
- 1 teaspoon cornstarch
- 1 teaspoon dry sherry
- 12 oz. beef, sliced into strips
- 1 teaspoon toasted sesame oil
- 2 tablespoons oyster sauce
- 1 lb. baby bok choy, sliced
- 3 tablespoons chicken broth

Directions:

1. Mix soy sauce, ginger, cornstarch and dry sherry in a bowl.
2. Toss the beef in the mixture.
3. Pour oil into a pan over medium heat.
4. Cook the beef for 5 minutes, stirring.
5. Add oyster sauce, bok choy and chicken broth to the pan.
6. Cook for 1 minute.

Nutrition:

- Calories 247
- Total Fat: 15.8g
- Saturated Fat: 4g
- Cholesterol: 69mg
- Sodium: 569mg
- Total Carbohydrate: 6.3g
- Dietary Fiber: 1.1g
- Protein: 25g

25. Grilled Pork with Salsa

Preparation Time: 30 minutes
Cooking Time: 15 minutes
Servings: 4
Ingredients:
Salsa

- 1 onion, chopped
- 1 tomato, chopped
- 1 peach, chopped
- 1 apricot, chopped
- 1 tablespoon olive oil
- 1 tablespoon lime juice
- 2 tablespoons fresh cilantro, chopped
- Salt and pepper to taste

Pork

- 1 lb. pork tenderloin, sliced
- 1 tablespoon olive oil
- Salt and pepper to taste
- ½ teaspoon ground cumin
- ¾ teaspoon chili powder

Directions:

1. Combine salsa ingredients in a bowl.
2. Cover and refrigerate.
3. Brush pork tenderloin with oil.
4. Season with salt, pepper, cumin and chili powder.
5. Grill pork for 5 to 7 minutes per side.
6. Slice pork and serve with salsa.

Nutrition:

- Calories: 219
- Total Fat: 9.5g
- Saturated Fat: 1.8g
- Cholesterol: 74mg
- Sodium: 512mg
- Total Carbohydrate: 8.3g
- Dietary Fiber: 1.5g
- Protein: 24g
- Total Sugars: 6g
- Potassium: 600mg

26. Chicken Pesto

Preparation Time: 15 minutes
Cooking Time: 25 minutes
Servings: 4
Ingredients:
- 1 lb. chicken cutlet
- Salt and pepper to taste
- 1 tablespoon olive oil
- ½ cup onion, chopped
- ½ cup heavy cream
- ½ cup dry white wine
- 1 tomato, chopped
- ¼ cup pesto
- 2 tablespoons basil, chopped

Directions:
1. Season chicken with salt and pepper.
2. Pour oil into a pan over medium heat.
3. Cook chicken for 3 to 4 minutes per side.
4. Place the chicken on a plate.
5. Add the onion to the pan.
6. Cook for 1 minute.
7. Stir in the rest of the ingredients.
8. Bring to a boil.
9. Simmer for 15 minutes.
10. Put the chicken back to the pan.
11. Cook for 2 more minutes and then serve.

Nutrition:
- Calories: 371
- Total Fat: 23.7g
- Saturated Fat: 9.2g
- Cholesterol: 117mg
- Sodium: 361mg
- Total Carbohydrate: 5.7g
- Dietary Fiber: 1g
- Protein: 27.7g
- Total Sugars: 3g
- Potassium: 567mg

27. Garlic Parmesan Chicken Wings

Preparation Time: 20 minutes
Cooking Time: 20 minutes
Servings: 8
Ingredients:

- Cooking spray
- ½ cup all-purpose flour
- Pepper to taste
- 2 tablespoons garlic powder
- 3 eggs, beaten
- 1 ¼ cups Parmesan cheese, grated
- 2 cups breadcrumbs
- 2 lb. chicken wings

Directions:

1. Preheat your oven to 450 degrees F.
2. Spray baking pan with oil.
3. In a bowl, mix the flour, pepper and garlic powder.
4. Add eggs to another bowl.
5. Mix the Parmesan cheese and breadcrumbs in another bowl.
6. Dip the chicken wings in the first, second and third bowls.
7. Spray chicken wings with oil.
8. Bake in the oven for 20 minutes.

Nutrition:

- Calories: 221
- Total Fat: 11.6g
- Saturated Fat: 3.9g
- Cholesterol: 122mg
- Sodium: 242mg
- Total Carbohydrate: 8g
- Dietary Fiber: 0.4g
- Protein: 16g
- Total Sugars: 3g
- Potassium: 163mg

28. Crispy Baked Shrimp

Preparation Time: 15 minutes
Cooking Time: 10 minutes
Servings: 4
Ingredients:

- ¼ cup whole-wheat breadcrumbs
- 3 tablespoons olive oil, divided
- 1 ½ lb. jumbo shrimp, peeled and deveined
- Salt and pepper to taste
- 2 tablespoons lemon juice
- 1 tablespoon garlic, chopped
- 2 tablespoons butter
- ¼ cup Parmesan cheese, grated
- 2 tablespoons chives, chopped

Directions:

1. Preheat your oven to 425 degrees F.
2. Add breadcrumbs to a pan over medium heat.
3. Cook until toasted.
4. Transfer to a plate.
5. Coat baking pan with 1 tablespoon oil.
6. Arrange shrimp in a single layer in a baking pan.
7. Season with salt and pepper.
8. Mix lemon juice, garlic and butter in a bowl.
9. Pour mixture on top of the shrimp.
10. Add Parmesan cheese and chives to the breadcrumbs.
11. Sprinkle breadcrumbs on top of the shrimp.
12. Bake for 10 minutes.

Nutrition:

- Calories: 340
- Total Fat: 18.7g
- Saturated Fat: 6g
- Cholesterol: 293mg
- Sodium: 374mg
- Total Carbohydrate: 6g
- Dietary Fiber: 0.8g
- Protein: 36.9g
- Total Sugars: 2g
- Potassium: 483mg

29. Herbed Mediterranean Fish Fillet

Preparation Time: 20 minutes
Cooking Time: 1 hour
Servings: 6
Ingredients:

- 3 lb. sea bass fillet
- Salt to taste
- 2 tablespoons tarragon, chopped
- ¼ cup dry white wine
- 3 tablespoons olive oil, divided
- 1 tablespoon butter
- 2 garlic cloves, minced
- 2 cups whole-wheat breadcrumbs
- 3 tablespoons parsley, chopped
- 3 tablespoons oregano, chopped
- 3 tablespoons fresh basil, chopped

Directions:

1. Preheat your oven to 350 degrees F.
2. Season fish with salt and tarragon.
3. Pour half of the oil into a roasting pan.
4. Stir in wine.
5. Add the fish in the roasting pan.
6. Bake in the oven for 50 minutes.
7. Add remaining oil to a pan over medium heat.
8. Cook herbs, breadcrumbs and salt.
9. Spread breadcrumb mixture on top of fish and bake for 5 minutes.

Nutrition:

- Calories: 288
- Total Fat: 12.7g
- Saturated Fat: 2.9g
- Cholesterol: 65mg
- Sodium: 499mg
- Total Carbohydrate: 10.4g
- Dietary Fiber: 1.8g
- Protein: 29.5g
- Total Sugars: 1g
- Potassium: 401mg

30. Mushroom Stuffed with Ricotta

Preparation Time: 10 minutes
Cooking Time: 10 minutes
Servings: 4
Ingredients:

- 4 large mushrooms, stemmed
- 1 tablespoon olive oil
- Salt and pepper to taste
- ¼ cup basil, chopped
- 1 cup ricotta cheese
- ¼ cup Parmesan cheese, grated

Directions:

1. Preheat your grill.
2. Coat the mushrooms with oil.
3. Season with salt and pepper.
4. Grill for 5 minutes.
5. Stuff each mushroom with a mixture of basil, ricotta cheese and Parmesan cheese.
6. Grill for another 5 minutes.

Nutrition:

- Calories: 259
- Total Fat: 17.3g
- Saturated Fat: 5.4g
- Cholesterol: 24mg
- Sodium: 509mg
- Total Carbohydrate: 14.9g
- Dietary Fiber: 2.6g
- Protein: 12.2g
- Total Sugars: 7g
- Potassium: 572mg

31. Thai Chopped Salad

Preparation Time: 15 minutes
Cooking Time: 0 minutes
Servings: 4
Ingredients:
- 10 oz. kale and cabbage mix
- 14 oz. tofu, sliced into cubes and fried crispy
- ½ cup vinaigrette

Directions:
1. Arrange kale and cabbage in a serving platter.
2. Top with the tofu cubes.
3. Drizzle with the vinaigrette.

Nutrition:
- Calories: 332
- Total Fat: 15g
- Saturated Fat: 1.5g
- Cholesterol: 0mg
- Sodium: 236mg
- Total Carbohydrate: 26.3g
- Dietary Fiber: 7.6g
- Protein: 1.3g
- Total Sugars: 13g
- Potassium: 41mg

32. Chicken Kurma

Preparation Time: 20 minutes
Cooking Time: 25 minutes
Servings: 6
Ingredients:

- 1 tablespoon olive oil
- 1 onion, diced
- 3 garlic cloves, sliced thinly
- 1 ginger, minced
- 2 tomatoes, diced
- 1 serrano pepper, minced
- Salt and pepper to taste
- 1 teaspoon ground turmeric
- 1 tablespoon tomato paste
- 1 ½ lb. chicken, sliced
- 1 red bell pepper, chopped

Directions:

1. Pour oil into a pan over medium heat.
2. Cook onion for 3 minutes.
3. Add garlic, ginger, tomatoes, Serrano pepper, salt, pepper, and turmeric and tomato paste.
4. Bring to a boil.
5. Reduce heat and simmer for 10 minutes.
6. Add chicken and cook for 5 minutes.
7. Stir in red bell pepper.
8. Cook for 5 minutes.

Nutrition:

- Calories: 175
- Total Fat: 15.2g
- Saturated Fat: 3g
- Cholesterol: 115mg
- Sodium: 400mg
- Total Carbohydrate: 7g
- Dietary Fiber: 1.8g
- Protein: 24g
- Total Sugars: 3g
- Potassium: 436mg

33. Green Chicken Curry

Preparation Time: 15 minutes
Cooking Time: 45 minutes
Servings: 4
Ingredients:

- 1 pound grass-fed skinless, boneless chicken breasts, cubed
- 1 tablespoon olive oil
- 2 tablespoons green curry paste
- 1 cup unsweetened coconut milk
- 1 cup homemade chicken broth
- 1 cup asparagus spears, trimmed and cut into pieces
- 1 cup green beans, trimmed and cut into pieces
- Salt and ground black pepper, to taste
- ¼ cup fresh basil leaves, chopped

Directions:

1. In a wok, heat the oil over medium heat and sauté the curry paste for about 1–2 minutes.
2. Add the chicken and cook for about 8–10 minutes.
3. Add coconut milk and broth and bring to a boil.
4. Adjust the heat low and cook for about 8–10 minutes.
5. Add the asparagus, green beans, salt, and black pepper, and cook for about 4–5 minutes or until desired doneness.
6. Serve hot.

Nutrition:

- Calories: 294
- Net Carbs: 4.3g
- Total Fat: 16.2g
- Saturated Fat: 9.6g
- Cholesterol: 66mg
- Sodium: 456mg
- Total Carbs: 6.4g
- Fiber: 2.1g
- Sugar: 3.6g
- Protein: 28.6g

34. Beef with Bell Peppers

Preparation Time: 15 minutes
Cooking Time: 25 minutes
Servings: 4
Ingredients:
- 1 tablespoon olive oil
- 1 pound grass-fed flank steak, cut into thin slices across the grain diagonally
- 1 red bell pepper, seeded and cut into thin strips
- 1 green bell pepper, seeded and cut into thin strips
- 1 tablespoon fresh ginger, minced
- 3 tablespoons low-sodium soy sauce
- 1½ tablespoons balsamic vinegar
- 2 teaspoons Sriracha

Directions:
1. In a large non-stick wok, heat the oil over medium-high heat and sear the steak slices for about 2 minutes.
2. Add bell peppers and cook for about 2-3 minutes, stirring continuously.
3. With a slotted spoon, transfer the beef mixture into a bowl.
4. In the wok, add the remaining ingredients over medium heat and bring to a boil.
5. Cook for about 1 minute, stirring frequently.
6. Add the beef mixture and cook for about 1-2 minutes.
7. Serve hot.

Nutrition:
- Calories: 274
- Net Carbs: 3.8g
- Total Fat: 13.1g
- Saturated Fat: 4.5g
- Cholesterol: 62mg
- Sodium: 744mg
- Total Carbs: 5g
- Fiber: 1.2g
- Sugar: 2.3g
- Protein: 32.9g

CHAPTER 13:

Poultry Recipes

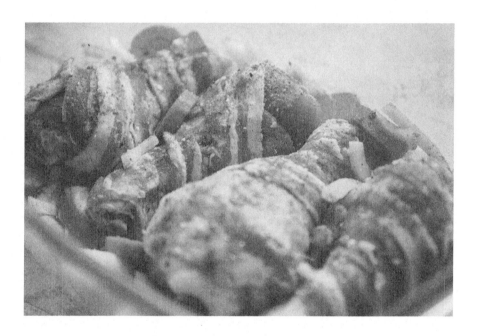

35. Egg Butter

Preparation Time: 5 minutes
Cooking Time: 0 minutes
Servings: 2
Ingredients:

- 2 large eggs, hard-boiled
- 3-ounce unsalted butter
- ½ teaspoon dried oregano
- ½ teaspoon dried basil
- 2 leaves of iceberg lettuce
- ½ teaspoon of sea salt
- ¼ teaspoon ground black pepper

Directions:

1. Peel the eggs, then chop them finely and place in a medium bowl.
2. Add remaining ingredients and stir well.
3. Serve egg butter wrapped in a lettuce leaf.

Nutrition:

- Calories: 159
- Fat: 16.5g
- Fiber: 0g
- Protein: 3g

36. Shredded Chicken in a Lettuce Wrap

Preparation Time: 5 minutes
Cooking Time: 15 minutes
Servings: 2
Ingredients:

- 2 leaves of iceberg lettuce
- 2 large chicken thigh
- 2 tablespoons shredded cheddar cheese
- 3 cups hot water
- 4 tablespoons tomato sauce
- 1 tablespoon soy sauce
- 1 tablespoon red chili powder
- ¾ teaspoon salt
- ½ teaspoon cracked black pepper

Directions:

1. Turn on your multicooker, place chicken thighs in it, and add remaining ingredients except for lettuce.
2. Stir until just mixed, shut the multicooker with a lid and cook for 15 minutes at high pressure and when done, release the pressure naturally.
3. Then open the multicooker, transfer chicken to a cutting board and shred with two forks.
4. Evenly divide the chicken between two lettuce leaves, and drizzle with some of the cooking liquid, reserving the remaining cooking liquid for later use as chicken broth.
5. Serve.

Nutrition:

- Calories: 143.5
- Fat: 1.4g
- Protein: 21.7g
- Carbs: 3.4g
- Fiber: 0.7g

37. Bacon-Wrapped Chicken Bites

Preparation Time: 10 minutes
Cooking Time: 20 minutes
Servings: 2
Ingredients:

- 1 chicken thigh, debone, cut into small pieces
- 4 slices of bacon, cut into thirds
- 2 tablespoons garlic powder
- ¼ teaspoon salt
- ½ teaspoon ground black pepper

Directions:

1. Turn on the oven, then set it to 400°F and let it preheat.
2. Cut chicken into small pieces, then place them in a bowl, add salt, garlic powder, and black pepper and toss until well coated.
3. Wrap each chicken piece with a bacon strip, place in a baking dish and bake for 15 to 20 minutes until crispy, turning carefully every 5 minutes.
4. Serve.

Nutrition:

- Calories: 153
- Fat: 8.7g
- Protein: 15g
- Carbs: 2.7g
- Fiber: 0.7g

38. Cheesy Bacon Wrapped Chicken

Preparation Time: 5 minutes
Cooking Time: 25 minutes
Servings: 2
Ingredients:
- 2 chicken thighs, boneless
- 2 strips of bacon
- 2 tablespoons shredded cheddar cheese
- 1/3 teaspoon salt
- 2/3 teaspoon paprika
- 1/4 teaspoon garlic powder

Directions:
1. Turn on the oven, then set it to 400°F and let it preheat.
2. Meanwhile, season chicken thighs with salt, paprika, and garlic on both sides, and then place them onto a baking sheet greased with oil.
3. Top each chicken thighs with a bacon strip and then bake for 15 to 20 minutes until the chicken has cooked through, and the bacon is crispy.
4. When done, sprinkle cheese over chicken, continue baking for 5 minutes until cheese has melted and golden, and then serve.

Nutrition:
- Calories: 172.5
- Fat: 11.5g
- Protein: 14.5g
- Carbs: 0.5g
- Fiber: 0.5g

39. Beans and Sausage

Preparation Time: 5 minutes
Cooking Time: 6 minutes
Servings: 2
Ingredients:
- 4 ounces green beans
- 4 ounces chicken sausage, sliced
- ½ teaspoon dried basil
- ½ teaspoon dried oregano
- 1/3 cup chicken broth, from chicken sausage
- 1 tablespoon avocado oil
- ¼ teaspoon salt
- 1/8 teaspoon ground black pepper

Directions:
1. Turn on your multicooker, place all the ingredients in its inner pot and shut with lid in the sealed position.
2. Press the "manual" button, cook for 6 minutes at high-pressure settings and when done, do quick pressure release.
3. Serve immediately.

Nutrition:
- Calories: 151
- Fat: 9.4g
- Protein: 11.7g
- Carbs: 3.4g
- Fiber: 1.6g

40. Paprika Rubbed Chicken

Preparation Time: 5 minutes
Cooking Time: 25 minutes
Servings: 2
Ingredients:

- 2 chicken thighs, boneless
- ¼ tablespoon fennel seeds, ground
- ½ teaspoon hot paprika
- ¼ teaspoon smoked paprika
- ½ teaspoon minced garlic
- ¼ teaspoon salt
- 2 tablespoons avocado oil

Directions:

1. Turn on the oven, then set it to 325°F and let it preheat.
2. Prepare the spice mix and for this, take a small bowl, add all the ingredients in it, except for chicken, and stir until well mixed.
3. Brush the mixture on all sides of the chicken, rub it well into the meat, then place chicken onto a baking sheet and roast for 15 to 25 minutes until thoroughly cooked, basting every 10 minutes with the drippings.
4. Serve.

Nutrition:

- Calories: 102.3
- Fat: 8g
- Protein: 7.2g
- Carbs: 0.3g
- Fiber: 0.5g

41. Teriyaki Chicken

Preparation Time: 5 minutes
Cooking Time: 18 minutes
Servings: 2
Ingredients:
- 2 chicken thighs, boneless
- 2 tablespoons soy sauce
- 1 tablespoon swerve sweetener
- 1 tablespoon avocado oil

Directions:
1. Take a skillet pan, place it over medium heat, add oil and when hot, add chicken thighs and cook for 5 minutes per side until seared.
2. Then sprinkle sugar over chicken thighs, drizzle with soy sauce and bring the sauce to boil.
3. Switch heat to medium-low level, continue cooking for 3 minutes until chicken is evenly glazed, and then transfer to a plate.
4. Serve chicken with cauliflower rice.

Nutrition:
- Calories: 150
- Fat: 9g
- Protein: 17.3g
- Carbs: 0.8g
- Fiber: 0.5g

42. Chili Lime Chicken with Coleslaw

Preparation Time: 35 minutes
Cooking Time: 8 minutes
Servings: 2
Ingredients:

- 1 chicken thigh, boneless
- 2 ounces coleslaw
- ¼ teaspoon minced garlic
- ¾ tablespoon apple cider vinegar
- ½ of a lime, juiced, zested
- ¼ teaspoon paprika
- ¼ teaspoon salt
- 2 tablespoons avocado oil
- 1 tablespoon unsalted butter

Directions:

1. Prepare the marinade and for this, take a medium bowl, add vinegar, oil, garlic, paprika, salt, lime juice, and zest and stir until well mixed.
2. Cut chicken thighs into bite-size pieces, toss until well mixed, and marinate it in the refrigerator for 30 minutes.
3. Then take a skillet pan, place it over medium-high heat, add butter and marinated chicken pieces and cook for 8 minutes until golden brown and thoroughly cooked.
4. Serve chicken with coleslaw.

Nutrition:

- Calories: 157.3
- Fat: 12.8g
- Protein: 9g
- Carbs: 1g
- Fiber: 0.5g

43. Lime Garlic Chicken Thighs

Preparation Time: 35 minutes
Cooking Time: 15 minutes
Servings: 2
Ingredients:
- 2 boneless chicken thighs, skinless
- ¾ teaspoon garlic powder
- 1 ½ teaspoon all-purpose seasoning
- ½ of lime, juiced, zested
- 1 ½ tablespoon avocado oil

Directions:
1. Take a medium bowl, place chicken in it, and sprinkle with garlic powder, all-purpose seasoning, and lime zest.
2. Drizzle with lime juice, toss until well coated and let chicken thighs marinate for 30 minutes.
3. Then take a medium skillet pan, place it over medium heat, add oil and when hot, place marinated chicken thighs in it and cook for 5 to 7 minutes per side until thoroughly cooked.
4. Serve.

Nutrition:
- Calories: 260
- Fat: 15.6g
- Protein: 26.8g
- Carbs: 1.3g
- Fiber: 0.6g

44. Bacon Ranch Deviled Eggs

Preparation Time: 5 minutes
Cooking Time: None
Servings: 2
Ingredients:
- 1 slice of bacon, chopped, cooked
- 2/3 teaspoons ranch dressing
- 1 ½ tablespoon mayonnaise
- 1/3 teaspoon mustard paste
- 2 eggs, boiled
- ¼ teaspoon paprika

Directions:
1. Peel the boiled eggs, then slice in half lengthwise and transfer egg yolks to a medium bowl by using a spoon.
2. Mash the egg yolk, add remaining ingredients, except for bacon and paprika and stir until well combined.
3. Pipe the egg yolk mixture into egg whites, sprinkle with bacon and paprika and then serve.

Nutrition:
- Calories: 260
- Fat: 24g
- Protein: 8.9g
- Carbs: 0.6g
- Fiber: 0.1g

45. Deviled Eggs with Mushrooms

Preparation Time: 5 minutes
Cooking Time: None
Servings: 2
Ingredients:

- 1 tablespoon chopped mushroom
- 2 teaspoons mayonnaise
- ½ teaspoon apple cider vinegar
- 1 teaspoon butter, unsalted
- 2 eggs, boiled
- ¼ teaspoon salt
- ¼ teaspoon ground black pepper
- ¼ teaspoon dried parsley

Directions:

1. Peel the boiled eggs, then slice in half lengthwise and transfer egg yolks to a medium bowl by using a spoon.
2. Mash the egg yolk, add remaining ingredients and stir until well combined.
3. Pipe the egg yolk mixture into egg whites, sprinkle with black pepper and then serve.

Nutrition:

- Calories: 130.5g
- Fats: 10.9g
- Protein: 7.1g
- Carbs: 0.6g
- Fiber: 0.1g

46. Chicken and Peanut Stir-Fry

Preparation Time: 5 minutes
Cooking Time: None
Servings: 2
Ingredients:

- 2 chicken thighs, cubed
- ½ cup broccoli florets
- ¼ cup peanuts
- 1 tablespoon sesame oil
- 1 ½ tablespoon soy sauce
- ½ teaspoon garlic powder

Directions:

1. Take a skillet pan, place it over medium heat, add ½ tablespoons oil and when hot, add chicken cubes and cook for 4 minutes until browned on all sides.
2. Then add broccoli florets and continue cooking for 2 minutes until tender-crisp.
3. Add remaining ingredients, stir well and cook for another 2 minutes.
4. Serve.

Nutrition:

- Calories: 266
- Fat: 19g
- Protein: 18.5g
- Carbs: 4g
- Fiber: 1.4g

47. Lemony Chicken Drumsticks

Preparation Time: 15 minutes
Cooking Time: 40-50 minutes
Servings: 6
Ingredients:
- 3 pounds grass-fed chicken drumsticks
- ½ cup butter, melted
- ¼ cup fresh lemon juice
- 2 teaspoons garlic, minced
- 2 teaspoons Italian seasoning
- Salt and ground white pepper, to taste

Directions:
1. Add butter, lemon juice, garlic, Italian seasoning, salt, and black pepper in a large mixing bowl and mix well.
2. Add the chicken drumsticks and coat with the marinade generously.
3. Cover the bowl and refrigerate for at least 3–5 hours.
4. Preheat the oven to 400°F.
5. Grease a large baking sheet.
6. Arrange the drumsticks onto the prepared baking sheet in a single layer.
7. Bake for approximately 40 minutes or until desired doneness.
8. Serve hot

Nutrition:
- Calories: 528
- Net Carbs: 0.6g
- Total Fat: 28.8g
- Saturated Fat: 13.3g
- Cholesterol: 241mg
- Sodium: 320mg
- Total Carbs: 0.7g
- Fiber: 0.1g
- Sugar: 0.4g
- Protein: 62.7g

48. Lemony Chicken Thighs

Preparation Time: 10 minutes
Cooking Time: 25 minutes
Servings: 4
Ingredients:

- 2 tablespoons olive oil, divided
- 1 tablespoon fresh lemon juice
- 1 tablespoon lemon zest, grated
- 2 teaspoons dried oregano
- 1 teaspoon dried thyme
- Salt and ground black pepper, to taste
- 1½ pounds grass-fed bone-in chicken thighs

Directions:

1. Preheat the oven to 420°F.
2. Add 1 tablespoon of the oil, lemon juice, lemon zest, dried herbs, salt, and black pepper in a large mixing bowl and mix well.
3. Add the chicken thighs and coat with the mixture generously.
4. Refrigerate to marinate for at least 20 minutes.
5. In an oven-proof wok, heat the remaining oil over medium-high heat and sear the chicken thighs for about 2-3 minutes per side.
6. Immediately, transfer the wok into the oven and bake for approximately 10 minutes.
7. Serve hot.

Nutrition:

- Calories: 388
- Net Carbs: 0.5g
- Total Fat: 19.7g
- Saturated Fat: 4.5g
- Cholesterol: 151mg
- Sodium: 186mg
- Total Carbs: 1g
- Fiber: 0.5g
- Sugar: 0.2g
- Protein: 49.4g

49. Turkey Meatloaf

Preparation Time: 15 minutes
Cooking Time: 40-50 minutes
Servings: 8
Ingredients:
Meatloaf

- 2 pounds ground turkey
- 1 cup cheddar cheese, shredded
- 1 tablespoon dried onion, minced
- 1 teaspoon dried garlic, minced
- 1 teaspoon garlic powder
- 1 teaspoon red chili powder
- 1 teaspoon ground mustard
- Salt, to taste
- 1 organic egg
- 2 ounces sugar-free BBQ sauce

Topping

- 2 ounces sugar-free BBQ sauce
- 5 cooked bacon slices, chopped
- ½ cup cheddar cheese, shredded

Directions:

1. Preheat the oven to 400°F.
2. Grease a 9x13-inch casserole dish.
3. For meatloaf: Add all ingredients in a mixing bowl and mix until well combined.
4. Place the mixture into the prepared casserole dish evenly and press to smooth the surface.
5. Coat the top of meatloaf with BBQ sauce evenly and sprinkle with bacon, followed by the cheese.
6. Bake for approximately 40 minutes.
7. Remove the meatloaf from the oven and place onto a wire rack to cool slightly.
8. Cut the meatloaf into desired sized slices and serve warm.

Nutrition:

- Calories: 380 Net Carbs: 6.4g Total Fat: 21.7g
- Saturated Fat: 6.9g Cholesterol: 175mg
- Sodium: 654mg Total Carbs: 6.6g Fiber: 0.2g
- Sugar: 2.8g Protein: 40.1g

CHAPTER 14:

Meat Recipes

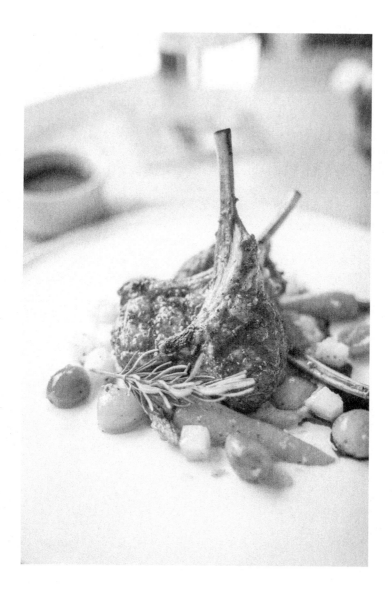

50. Beef and Broccoli Stir-Fry

Preparation Time: 20 minutes
Cooking Time: 15 minutes
Servings: 4
Ingredients:
- ¼ cup soy sauce
- 1 tablespoon sesame oil
- 1 teaspoon garlic chili paste
- 1 pound beef sirloin
- 2 tablespoons almond flour
- 2 tablespoons coconut oil
- 2 cups chopped broccoli florets
- 1 tablespoon grated ginger
- 3 garlic cloves, minced

Directions:
1. Whisk together the soy sauce, sesame oil, and chili paste in a small bowl.
2. Slice the beef and toss with almond flour, then place in a plastic freezer bag.
3. Pour in the sauce and toss to coat, then let rest for 20 minutes.
4. Heat the oil in a large skillet over medium-high heat.
5. Pour the beef and sauce into the skillet and cook until the beef is browned.
6. Push the beef to the sides of the skillet and add the broccoli, ginger, and garlic.
7. Sauté until the broccoli is tender-crisp, then toss it all together and serve hot.

Nutrition:
- Calories: 350
- Fat: 19g
- Protein: 37.5g
- Carbs: 6.5g
- Fiber: 2g

51. Rosemary Roasted Pork with Cauliflower

Preparation Time: 10 minutes
Cooking Time: 20 minutes
Servings: 4
Ingredients:

- 1 ½ pound boneless pork tenderloin
- 1 tablespoon coconut oil
- 1 tablespoon fresh chopped rosemary
- Salt and pepper
- 1 tablespoon olive oil
- 2 cups cauliflower florets

Directions:

1. Rub the pork with coconut oil, then season with rosemary, salt, and pepper.
2. Heat the olive oil in a large skillet over medium-high heat.
3. Add the pork and cook for 2 to 3 minutes on each side until browned.
4. Sprinkle the cauliflower in the skillet around the pork.
5. Reduce the heat to low, then cover the skillet and cook for 8 to 10 minutes until the pork is cooked through.
6. Slice the pork and serve with the cauliflower.

Nutrition:

- Calories: 300
- Fat: 15.5g
- Protein: 37g
- Carbs: 3g
- Fiber: 1.5g

52. Sweet & Sour Pork

Preparation Time: 15 minutes
Cooking Time: 15 minutes
Servings: 4
Ingredients:
- 1 lb. pork chops
- Salt and pepper to taste
- ½ cup sesame seeds
- 2 tablespoons peanut oil
- 2 tablespoons soy sauce
- 3 tablespoons apricot jam

Directions:
1. Season pork chops with salt and pepper.
2. Press sesame seeds on both sides of pork.
3. Pour oil into a pan over medium heat.
4. Cook pork for 3 to 5 minutes per side.
5. Transfer to a plate.
6. In a bowl, mix soy sauce and apricot jam.
7. Simmer for 3 minutes.
8. Pour sauce over the pork before serving.

Nutrition:
- Calories: 414 Fat: 27.5g Carbs: 12.9g Fiber: 1.8g Protein: 29g

53. Garlic Pork Loin

Preparation Time: 15 minutes
Cooking Time: 1 hour
Servings: 6
Ingredients:
- 1 ½ lb. pork loin roast
- 4 garlic cloves, sliced into slivers
- Salt and pepper to taste

Directions:
1. Preheat your oven to 425°F:
2. Make several slits all over the pork roast.
3. Insert garlic slivers. Sprinkle with salt and pepper.
4. Roast in the oven for 1 hour.

Nutrition:
- Calories: 235 Fat: 13.3g Carbs: 1.7g Fiber: 0.3g Protein: 25.7g

54. Keto Grilled Lamb Steaks

Preparation Time: 20 minutes (+ 4 hours marinating time)
Cooking Time: 10 minutes
Servings: 4
Ingredients:

- 4 bone-in lamb leg steaks
- ¼ cup lime juice
- ¼ cup orange juice
- ¼ chopped fresh cilantro
- 4 minced garlic cloves
- 1 minced jalapeno pepper
- 1 tablespoon brown sugar
- 1 tablespoon cumin
- 1 dried oregano
- ½ tablespoon salt
- ½ tablespoon pepper

Avocado Sauce:

- 1 avocado, peeled, pitted and chopped
- 2 tablespoons chopped red onion
- 1 tablespoon lime juice
- 1 tablespoon chopped fresh cilantro
- 1/4 teaspoons cumin
- Pinch each salt and pepper

Directions:

1. First, Whisk together lime and orange juice, garlic, cilantro, jalapeno, cumin, oregano, brown sugar salt and pepper.
2. Pour over lamb in a resalable plastic sack, seal and refrigerate for at least 4 hours.
3. Preheat grill to medium-high heat and oil grind well. Now grill steaks, turning once, for around 7 minutes or until wanted doneness.
4. In the meantime, mix avocado, red onion, cilantro, cumin, lime juice pepper and salt.
5. Serve with steaks.

Nutrition:

- Calories: 320 Fat: 19g Protein: 37.5g
- Carbs: 3.7g Fiber: 2g

55. Steak with Pesto

Preparation Time: 10 minutes
Cooking Time: 10 minutes
Servings: 4
Ingredients:
- 1 tablespoon butter
- 4 (6-ounce) grass-fed flank steaks
- Salt and ground black pepper, to taste
- ½ cup pesto

Directions:
1. For steak: In a wok, melt the butter over medium-high heat and cook steaks with salt and black pepper for about 3-5 minutes per side.
2. Transfer the steaks onto serving plates and serve with the topping of pesto.

Nutrition:
- Calories: 490
- Net Carbs: 1.5g
- Total Fat: 30g
- Saturated Fat: 10.2g
- Cholesterol: 109mg
- Sodium: 344mg
- Total Carbs: 2g
- Fiber: 0.5g
- Sugar: 2g
- Protein: 50.4g

56. Herbed Lamb Chops

Preparation Time: 10 minutes
Cooking Time: 20 minutes
Servings: 4
Ingredients:
- 1½ pounds grass-fed lamb loin chops, trimmed
- 1 tablespoon fresh lemon juice
- ¼ cup fresh parsley, chopped
- 2 tablespoons fresh mint leaves, chopped
- 1 tablespoon olive oil
- Salt and ground black pepper, to taste

Directions:
1. Preheat grill to medium-high heat. Grease the grill grate.
2. In a bowl, add lamb loin chops, lemon juice, parsley, mint, oil, salt, and black pepper and mix well.
3. Place the chops onto the grill and cook for about 10 minutes per side or until desired doneness.
4. Serve hot.

Nutrition:
- Calories: 350
- Net Carbs: 0.3g
- Total Fat: 16.1g
- Saturated Fat: 5g
- Cholesterol: 153mg
- Sodium: 172mg
- Total Carbs: 0.6g
- Fiber: 0.3g
- Sugar: 0.1g
- Protein: 48g

57. Grilled Pork Chops

Preparation Time: 10 minutes
Cooking Time: 12 minutes
Servings: 4
Ingredients:
- ¼ cup fresh basil leaves, minced
- 2 garlic cloves, minced
- 2 tablespoons butter, melted
- 2 tablespoons fresh lemon juice
- Salt and ground black pepper, as required
- 4 (6- to 8-ounce) bone-in pork loin chops

Directions:
1. In a baking dish, add the basil, garlic, butter, lemon juice, salt, and black pepper, and mix well.
2. Add the chops and generously coat with the mixture.
3. Cover the baking dish and refrigerate for about 30–45 minutes.
4. Preheat a gas grill to medium-high heat. Lightly, grease the grill grate.
5. Place chops onto the grill and cook for about 6 minutes per side or until desired doneness.
6. Serve hot.

Nutrition:
- Calories: 600
- Net Carbs: 0.6g
- Total Fat: 48.1g
- Saturated Fat: 19.6g
- Cholesterol: 162mg
- Sodium: 201mg
- Total Carbs: 0.7g
- Fiber: 0.1g
- Sugar: 0.2g
- Protein: 38.5g

CHAPTER 15:

Seafood & Fish Recipes

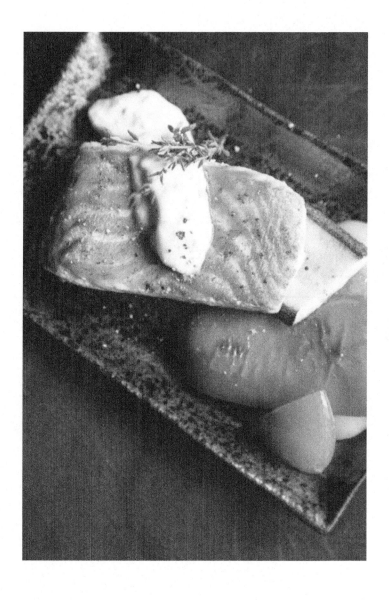

58. Crab Salad

Preparation Time: 10 minutes
Cooking Time: 10 minutes
Servings: 6
Ingredients:

- 8 oz. crab meat
- 2 celery stalks, sliced
- ½ tsp Worcestershire sauce
- ½ tsp old bay spice
- ½ tsp dried dill
- 1 tsp lemon juice
- 2 tbsp. fresh parsley, chopped
- ¼ cup mayonnaise
- ½ cup sour cream
- 4 oz. cream cheese
- 1 tbsp. garlic, crushed
- ¼ cup onion, diced
- 2 tbsp. butter

Directions:

1. Melt butter on a small pan over medium heat.
2. Add onion and sauté until softened.
3. Add garlic and sauté for a moment.
4. Transfer onion-garlic mixture to the massive bowl.
5. Add remaining ingredients to the bowl and stir everything well to mix.
6. Serve and luxuriate in.

Nutrition:

- Calories: 219
- Fat: 18.4g
- Carbohydrates: 5.6g
- Sugar: 1.1g
- Protein: 7.2g
- Cholesterol: 62mg

59. Easy Seafood Salad

Preparation Time: 10 minutes
Cooking Time: 3 minutes
Servings: 4
Ingredients:

- 8 oz. shrimp
- 8 oz. crab meat
- 1 tbsp. dill, chopped
- ½ cup mayonnaise
- 2 tsp lemon juice
- ¼ tsp old bay seasoning
- ¼ cup onion, minced
- ½ cup celery, chopped
- 1 lemon, quartered
- Pepper Salt

Directions:

1. Add lemon and water to the pot and convey to boil.
2. Add shrimp to the pot and cook for 1-2 minutes.
3. Drain shrimp well and place it on a large bowl.
4. Add remaining ingredients to the bowl and stir until well combined.
5. Cover salad bowl and place within the refrigerator for two hours.
6. Serve chilled and luxuriate in.

Nutrition:

- Calories: 240
- Fat: 11g
- Carbohydrates: 10g
- Sugar: 2.4g
- Protein: 20.6g
- Cholesterol: 157mg

60. Easy Crab Cakes

Preparation Time: 10 minutes
Cooking Time: 10 minutes
Servings: 2
Ingredients:
- 8 oz. crab meat
- 2 tbsp. butter
- ¼ tsp pepper
- ½ tsp old bay seasoning
- 2 tbsp. mayonnaise
- 1 egg, lightly beaten
- ¼ cup almond flour
- ¼ cup red pepper, diced
- 1 small onion, diced

Directions:
1. Add all ingredients except butter on a bowl and blend until well combined.
2. Make small patties from bowl mixture. Melt butter during a pan over medium heat.
3. Fry crab cakes for 2-3 minutes on all sides or until lightly golden brown.
4. Serve and luxuriate in.

Nutrition:
- Calories: 311
- Fat: 20.7g
- Carbohydrates: 10.3g
- Sugar: 3.4g
- Protein: 17.8g
- Cholesterol: 177mg

61. Nutritious Tuna Patties

Preparation Time: 10 minutes
Cooking Time: 15 minutes
Servings: 8
Ingredients:

- 2 cans tuna, drained and flaked
- 4 tbsp. olive oil
- ¼ cup fresh parsley, chopped
- 2 eggs, lightly beaten
- 3 garlic cloves, minced
- 2 tbsp. Dijon mustard
- 2 tbsp. mayonnaise
- ¼ tsp pepper
- ½ tsp salt

Directions:

1. Preheat the oven to 170°F.
2. In a bowl, mix tuna, parsley, eggs, garlic, Dijon mustard, mayonnaise, pepper, and salt.
3. Heat oil during a pan over medium heat.
4. Make small patties from tuna mixture and fry until golden brown, about 2-3 minutes per side.
5. Serve and luxuriate in.

Nutrition:

- Calories: 178
- Fat: 13.1g
- Carbohydrates: 1.7g
- Sugar: 0.4g
- Protein: 13.5g
- Cholesterol: 56mg

62. Quick Butter Cod

Preparation Time: 10 minutes
Cooking Time: 5 minutes
Servings: 4
Ingredients:
- 1 ½ lbs. cod fillets, cut into pieces
- ½ tsp paprika
- ¼ tsp ground pepper
- ¼ tsp garlic powder
- 6 tbsp. butter
- ½ tsp salt

Directions:
1. On a small bowl, mix paprika, pepper, garlic powder, and salt.
2. Coat fish pieces with seasoning mixture.
3. Melt 2 tbsp. of butter during a large pan over medium-high heat.
4. Add fish pieces to the pan and cook for two minutes.
5. Turn heat to medium. Add remaining butter on top of fish pieces and cook for 3-4 minutes.
6. Once fish is cooked thoroughly, then remove the pan from heat.
7. Add juice and stir well.
8. Serve and luxuriate in.

Nutrition:
- Calories: 291
- Fat: 18.8g
- Carbohydrates: 0.4g
- Sugar: 0.1g
- Protein: 30.6g
- Cholesterol: 129mg

63. Baked Tilapia

Preparation Time: 10 minutes
Cooking Time: 10 minutes
Servings: 4
Ingredients:

- 4 tilapia fillets
- 1 lemon zest
- 2 tbsp. fresh lemon juice
- 1 tbsp. garlic, minced
- ¼ cup butter, melted
- 2 tbsp. fresh parsley, chopped
- Pepper Salt

Directions:

1. Preheat the oven to 425°F.
2. On a small bowl, mix butter, lemon peel, juice, and garlic and put aside.
3. Season fish fillets with pepper and salt.
4. Place fish fillets onto the baking dish. Pour butter mixture over fish fillets.
5. Bake fish in a preheated oven for 10-12 minutes.
6. Garnish with parsley and serve.

Nutrition:

- Calories: 247
- Fat: 13.6g
- Carbohydrates: 1g
- Sugar: 0.2g
- Protein: 32.4g
- Cholesterol: 116mg

64. Shrimp Avocado Salad

Preparation Time: 10 minutes
Cooking Time: 5 minutes
Servings: 4
Ingredients:
- 16 oz. shrimp, thawed and drained
- 1 avocado, pitted and diced
- ¼ cup celery, chopped
- 1 small onion, chopped
- 2½ tbsp. fresh dill, chopped
- 1 tbsp. vinegar
- 1 tsp Dijon mustard
- ½ cup mayonnaise
- Pepper Salt

Directions:
1. On a small bowl, mix mayonnaise, dill, vinegar, and mustard. Set aside.
2. Add shrimp, onion, and celery during a bowl.
3. Pour mayonnaise mixture over shrimp and stir well.
4. Cover and place within the refrigerator for 1-2 hours.
5. Add avocado and serve immediately.

Nutrition:
- Calories: 279
- Fat: 13.1g
- Carbohydrates: 12.5g
- Sugar: 2.7g
- Protein: 27g
- Cholesterol: 246mg

65. Paprika Shrimp

Preparation Time: 10 minutes
Cooking Time: 50 minutes
Servings: 8
Ingredients:

- 2 lbs. shrimp, peeled and deveined
- 1 tsp paprika
- 5 garlic cloves, sliced
- 3/4 cup olive oil
- 1/2 tsp red pepper flakes, crushed
- 1/4 tsp pepper
- 1 tsp kosher salt

Directions:

1. Add oil, red pepper flakes, pepper, paprika, garlic, and salt into the slow cooker and stir well.
2. Cover and cook on high for a half-hour.
3. Add shrimp. Stir and cook for 10 minutes.
4. Cover again and cook for 10 minutes more.
5. Serve and luxuriate in.

Nutrition:

- Calories: 300
- Fat: 20.2g
- Carbohydrates: 2.7g
- Sugar: 0.3g
- Protein: 25g
- Cholesterol: 240mg

66. Zingy Lemon Fish

Preparation Time: 50 minutes
Cooking Time: 40 minutes
Servings: 4
Ingredients:
- 14 ounces fresh Gurnard fish fillets
- 2 tablespoons lemon juice
- 6 tablespoons butter
- ½ cup fine almond flour
- 2 teaspoons dried chives
- 1 teaspoon garlic powder
- 2 teaspoons dried dill
- 2 teaspoons onion powder
- Salt and pepper to taste

Directions:
1. Add almond flour, dried herbs, salt, and spices on a large plate and stir until well combined. Spread it all over the plate evenly.
2. Place a large pan over medium-high heat. Add half the butter and half the lemon juice. When butter just melts, place fillets on the pan and cook for 3 minutes. Move the fillets around the pan so that it absorbs the butter and lemon juice.
3. Add the remaining half butter and lemon juice. When butter melts, flip sides and cook the other side for 3 minutes.
4. Serve fillets with any butter remaining in the pan.

Nutrition:
- Calories 406
- Fat: 30.3g
- Protein: 29g
- Carbs: 3.5g
- Fiber: 0.7g

67. Keto Thai Fish with Curry and Coconut

Preparation Time: 50 minutes
Cooking Time: 40 minutes
Servings: 4
Ingredients:

- 25 ounces salmon (slice into bite-sized pieces)
- 15 ounces cauliflower (bite-sized florets)
- 14 ounces coconut cream
- 1-ounce olive oil
- 4 tablespoons butter
- Salt and pepper, to taste

Directions:

1. Preheat the oven to 400°F.
2. Sprinkle salt and pepper over the salmon generously. Toss it once, if possible.
3. Place the butter generously over all the salmon pieces and set aside.
4. Pour this cream mixture over the fish in the baking tray.
5. Meanwhile, boil the cauliflower florets in salted water for 5 minutes, strain and mash the florets coarsely. Set aside.
6. Transfer the creamy fish to a plate and serve with mashed cauliflower. Enjoy!

Nutrition:

- Calories: 880
- Fat: 75g
- Protein: 43g
- Carb: 9 g
- Fiber: 4g

68. Creamy Mackerel

Preparation Time: 10 minutes
Cooking Time: 20 minutes
Servings: 4
Ingredients:

- 2 shallots, minced
- 2 spring onions, chopped
- 2 tablespoons olive oil
- 4 mackerel fillets, skinless and cut into medium cubes
- 1 cup heavy cream
- 1 teaspoon cumin, ground
- ½ teaspoon oregano, dried
- A pinch of salt and black pepper
- 2 tablespoons chives, chopped

Directions:

1. Heat a pan with the oil over medium heat, add the spring onions and the shallots, stir and sauté for 5 minutes.
2. Add the fish and cook it for 4 minutes.
3. Add the rest of the ingredients, bring to a simmer, cook everything for 10 minutes more, divide between plates, and serve.

Nutrition:

- Calories: 403
- Fat: 33.9g
- Fiber: 0.4g
- Carbs: 2.7g
- Protein: 22g

69. Lime Mackerel

Preparation Time: 10 Minutes
Cooking Time: 30 Minutes
Servings: 4
Ingredients:
- 4 mackerel fillets, boneless
- 2 tablespoons lime juice
- 2 tablespoons olive oil
- A pinch of salt and black pepper
- ½ teaspoon sweet paprika

Directions:
1. Arrange the mackerel on a baking sheet lined with parchment paper, add the oil and the other ingredients, rub gently, introduce in the oven at 360°F and bake for 30 minutes.
2. Divide the fish between plates and serve.

Nutrition:
- Calories: 297 Fat: 22.7g Fiber 0.2g Carbs: 2g Protein: 21.1g

70. Turmeric Tilapia

Preparation Time: 10 minutes
Cooking Time: 12 minutes
Servings: 4
Ingredients:
- 4 tilapia fillets, boneless
- 2 tablespoons olive oil
- 1 teaspoon turmeric powder
- A pinch of salt and black pepper
- 2 spring onions, chopped
- ¼ teaspoon basil, dried
- ¼ teaspoon garlic powder
- 1 tablespoon parsley, chopped

Directions:
1. Heat a pan with the oil over medium heat, add the spring onions and cook them for 2 minutes.
2. Add the fish, turmeric, and the other ingredients, cook for 5 minutes on each side, divide between plates and serve.

Nutrition:
- Calories: 205 Fat: 8.6g Fiber: 0.4g Carbs: 1.1g Protein: 31.8g

71. Walnut Salmon Mix

Preparation Time: 10 Minutes
Cooking Time: 14 Minutes
Servings: 4
Ingredients:
- 4 salmon fillets, boneless
- 2 tablespoons avocado oil
- A pinch of salt and black pepper
- 1 tablespoon lime juice
- 2 shallots, chopped
- 2 tablespoons walnuts, chopped
- 2 tablespoons parsley, chopped

Directions:
1. Heat a pan with the oil over medium-high heat, add the shallots, stir and sauté for 2 minutes.
2. Add the fish and the other ingredients, cook for 6 minutes on each side, divide between plates and serve.

Nutrition:
- Calories 276
- Fat: 14.2g
- Fiber: 0.7g
- Carbs: 2.7g
- Protein: 35.8g

CHAPTER 16:

Salad Recipes

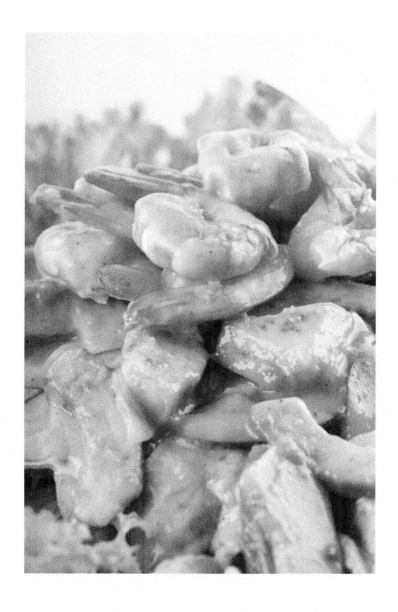

72. Bacon Avocado Salad

Preparation Time: 20 Minutes
Cooking Time: 0 Minutes
Servings: 4
Ingredients:
- 2 hard-boiled eggs, chopped
- 2 cups spinach
- 2 large avocados, 1 chopped and 1 sliced
- 2 small lettuce heads, chopped
- 1 spring onion, sliced
- 4 cooked bacon slices, crumbled

Directions:
1. In a large bowl, mix the eggs, spinach, avocados, lettuce, and onion. Set aside.
2. Make the vinaigrette: In a separate bowl, add the olive oil, mustard, and apple cider vinegar. Mix well.
3. Pour the vinaigrette into the large bowl and toss well.
4. Serve topped with bacon slices and sliced avocado.

Nutrition:
- Calories: 268Cal
- Fat: 16.9g
- Carbs: 8g
- Protein: 5g
- Fiber: 3g

73. Cauliflower and Cashew Nut Salad

Preparation Time: 10 Minutes
Cooking Time: 5 Minutes
Servings: 4
Ingredients:

- 1 head cauliflower, cut into florets
- ½ cup black olives, pitted and chopped
- 1 cup roasted bell peppers, chopped
- 1 red onion, sliced
- ½ cup cashew nuts
- Chopped celery leaves, for garnish

Directions:

1. Add the cauliflower into a pot of boiling salted water. Allow to boil for 4 to 5 minutes until fork-tender but still crisp.
2. Remove from the heat and drain on paper towels, then transfer the cauliflower to a bowl.
3. Add the olives, bell pepper, and red onion. Stir well.
4. Make the dressing: In a separate bowl, mix the olive oil, mustard, vinegar, salt, and pepper. Pour the dressing over the veggies and toss to combine.
5. Serve topped with cashew nuts and celery leaves.

Nutrition:

- Calories: 298Cal
- Fat: 20g
- Carbs: 4g
- Protein: 8g
- Fiber: 3g

74. Salmon and Lettuce Salad

Preparation Time: 10 Minutes
Cooking Time: 0 Minutes
Servings: 4
Ingredients:
- 1 tablespoon extra-virgin olive oil
- 2 slices smoked salmon, chopped
- 3 tablespoons mayonnaise
- 1 tablespoon lime juice
- Sea salt, to taste
- 1 cup romaine lettuce, shredded
- 1 teaspoon onion flakes
- ½ avocado, sliced

Directions:
1. In a bowl, stir together the olive oil, salmon, mayo, lime juice, and salt. Stir well until the salmon is coated fully.
2. Divide evenly the romaine lettuce and onion flakes among four serving plates. Spread the salmon mixture over the lettuce, then serve topped with avocado slices.

Nutrition:
- Calories: 271Cal
- Fat: 18g
- Carbs: 4g
- Protein: 6g
- Fiber: 3g

75. Prawns Salad with Mixed Lettuce Greens

Preparation Time: 10 Minutes
Cooking Time: 3 Minutes
Servings: 4
Ingredients:

- ½ pound (227 g) prawns, peeled and deveined
- Salt and chili pepper, to taste
- 1 tablespoon olive oil
- 2 cups mixed lettuce greens

Directions:

1. In a bowl, add the prawns, salt, and chili pepper. Toss well.
2. Warm the olive oil over medium heat. Add the seasoned prawns and fry for about 6 to 8 minutes, stirring occasionally, or until the prawns are opaque.
3. Remove from the heat and set the prawns aside on a platter.
4. Make the dressing: In a small bowl, mix the mustard, aioli, and lemon juice until creamy and smooth.
5. Make the salad: In a separate bowl, add the mixed lettuce greens. Pour the dressing over the greens and toss to combine.
6. Divide the salad among four serving plates and serve it alongside the prawns.

Nutrition:

- Calories: 228Cal
- Fat: 17g
- Carbs: 3g
- Protein: 5g
- Fiber: 8g

76. Shrimp, Tomato, and Avocado Salad

Preparation Time: 5 Minutes
Cooking Time: 30 Minutes
Servings: 4
Ingredients:
- 1 pound (454 g) shrimp, shelled and deveined
- 2 tomatoes, cubed
- 2 avocados, peeled and cubed
- A handful of fresh cilantro, chopped
- 4 green onions, minced
- Juice of 1 lime or lemon
- 1 tablespoon macadamia nut or avocado oil
- Celtic sea salt and fresh ground black pepper, to taste

Directions:
1. Combine the shrimp, tomatoes, avocados, cilantro, and onions in a large bowl.
2. Squeeze the lemon juice over the vegetables in the large bowl, then drizzle with avocado oil and sprinkle the salt and black pepper to season. Toss to combine well.
3. You can cover the salad, and refrigerate to chill for 45 minutes or serve immediately.

Nutrition:
- Calories: 158Cal
- Fat: 10g
- Carbs: 4g
- Protein: 9g
- Fiber: 3g

CHAPTER 17:

Soup and Stews

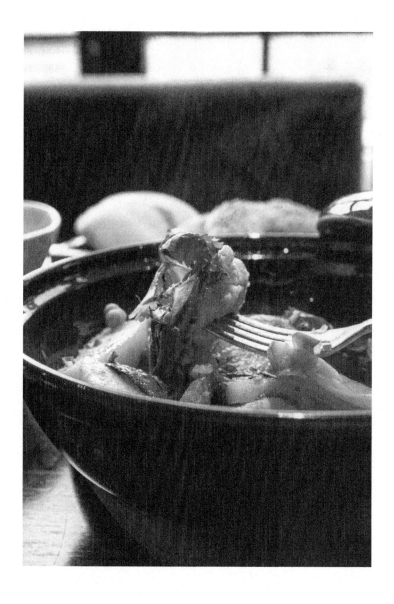

77. Hearty Fall Stew

Preparation Time: 15 minutes
Cooking Time: 8 hrs.
Servings: 6
Ingredients:
- 3 tablespoons extra-virgin olive oil, divided
- 1 (2-pound / 907-g) beef chuck roast, cut into 1-inch chunks
- 1/2 teaspoon salt
- 1/4 teaspoon freshly ground black pepper
- 1/4 cup apple cider vinegar
- 1/2 sweet onion, chopped
- 1 cup diced tomatoes
- 1 teaspoon dried thyme
- 11/2 cups pumpkin, cut into 1-inch chunks
- 2 cups beef broth
- 2 teaspoons minced garlic
- 1 tablespoon chopped fresh parsley, for garnish

Directions:
1. Add the beef to the skillet, and sprinkle salt and pepper to season.
2. Cook the beef for 7 minutes or until well browned.
3. Put the cooked beef into the slow cooker and add the remaining ingredients, except for the parsley, to the slow cooker. Stir to mix well.
4. Slow cook for 8 hrs. And top with parsley before serving.

Nutrition:
- Calories: 462
- Fat: 19.1g
- Fiber: 11.6g
- Carbohydrates: 10.7 g
- Protein: 18.6 g

78. Chicken Mushroom Soup

Preparation Time: 15 minutes
Cooking Time: 10-15 minutes
Servings: 4
Ingredients:

- 6 cups of chicken stock
- 5 slices of chopped bacon
- 4 cups cooked chicken breast, chopped
- 3 cups of water
- 2 cups of chopped celery root
- 2 cups of sliced yellow squash
- 2 tablespoons of olive oil
- 1/2 teaspoon of avocado oil
- 1/4 cup of chopped basil
- 1/4 cup of chopped onion
- 1/4 cup of chopped tomatoes
- 1 tablespoon of ground garlic
- 1 cup of sliced white mushrooms
- 1 cup green beans
- Salt
- Black pepper

Directions:

1. Heat oil in a skillet, add in half of the onions, sauté until soft.
2. Put in bacon and fry for a minute and a half.
3. Then, add in onions, garlic, tomatoes, and mushrooms, stir fry for three minutes.
4. Put in stock and fat water with the rest of the ingredients. Let it simmer for 10-15 minutes. Serve hot.

Nutrition:

- Calories: 268
- Fat: 10.5g
- Fiber: 4.9g
- Carbohydrates: 3.1 g
- Protein: 12.9g

79. Cold Green Beans and Avocado Soup

Preparation Time: 15 minutes
Cooking Time: 15 minutes
Servings: 4
Ingredients:

- 1 tbsp. butter
- 2 tbsp. almond oil
- 1 garlic clove, minced
- 1 cup (227 g) green beans (fresh or frozen)
- 1/4 avocado
- 1 cup heavy cream
- 1/2 cup grated cheddar cheese + extra for garnish
- 1/2 tsp. coconut aminos
- Salt to taste

Directions:

1. Heat the butter and almond oil in a large skillet and sauté the garlic for 30 seconds.
2. Add the green beans and stir-fry for 10 minutes or until tender.
3. Add the mixture to a food processor and top with the avocado, heavy cream, cheddar cheese, coconut aminos, and salt.
4. Blend the ingredients until smooth.
5. Pour the soup into serving bowls, cover with plastic wraps and chill in the fridge for at least 2 hours.
6. Enjoy afterward with a garnish of grated white sharp cheddar cheese

Nutrition:

- Calories: 301
- Fat: 3.1g
- Fiber: 11.5g
- Carbohydrates: 2.8 g
- Protein: 3.1g

80. Creamy Mixed Seafood Soup

Preparation Time: 15 minutes
Cooking Time: 15 minutes
Servings: 4
Ingredients:

- 1 tbsp. avocado oil
- 2 garlic cloves, minced
- 3/4 tbsp. almond flour
- 1 cup vegetable broth
- 1 tsp. dried dill
- 1 lb. frozen mixed seafood
- Salt and black pepper to taste
- 1 tbsp. plain vinegar
- 2 cups cooking cream
- Fresh dill leaves to garnish

Directions:

1. Heat oil sauté the garlic for 30 seconds or until fragrant.
2. Stir in the almond flour until brown.
3. Mix in the vegetable broth until smooth and stir in the dill, seafood mix, salt, and black pepper.
4. Bring the soup to a boil and then simmer for 3 to 4 minutes or until the seafood cooks.
5. Add the vinegar, cooking cream, and stir well. Garnish with dill, serve.

Nutrition:

- Calories: 361
- Fat: 12.4g
- Fiber: 8.5g
- Carbohydrates: 3.9 g
- Protein: 11.7g

81. Roasted Tomato and Cheddar Soup

Preparation Time: 10 minutes
Cooking Time: 15-20 minutes
Servings: 4
Ingredients:

- 2 tbsp. butter
- 2 medium yellow onions, sliced
- 4 garlic cloves, minced
- 5 thyme sprigs
- 8 basil leaves + extra for garnish
- 8 tomatoes
- 1/2 tsp. red chili flakes
- 2 cups vegetable broth
- Salt and black pepper to taste
- 1 cup grated cheddar cheese (white and sharp)

Directions:

1. Melt the butter in a pot and sauté the onions and garlic for 3 minutes or until softened.
2. Stir in the thyme, basil, tomatoes, red chili flakes, and vegetable broth.
3. Season with salt and black pepper.
4. Boil it then simmer for 10 minutes or until the tomatoes soften.
5. Puree all ingredients until smooth. Season.
6. Garnish with the cheddar cheese and basil. Serve warm.

Nutrition:

- Calories: 341
- Fat: 12.9g
- Fiber: 9.6g
- Carbohydrates: 4.8 g
- Protein: 4.1g

82. Healthy Celery Soup

Preparation Time: 10 minutes
Cooking Time: 20 minutes
Servings: 4
Ingredients:

- 3 cups celery, chopped
- 1 cup vegetable broth
- 5 oz. cream cheese
- 1 1/2 tbsp. fresh basil, chopped
- 1/4 cup onion, chopped
- 1 tbsp. garlic, chopped
- 1 tbsp. olive oil
- 1/4 tsp. pepper
- 1/2 tsp. salt

Directions:

1. Heat some oil.
2. Add celery, onion and garlic to the saucepan and sauté for 4-5 minutes or until softened.
3. Add broth and bring to boil. Turn heat to low and simmer.
4. Add basil and cream cheese and stir until cheese is melted.
5. Season soup with pepper and salt.
6. Puree the soup until smooth.
7. Serve and enjoy.

Nutrition:

- Calories: 201
- Fat: 5.4g
- Fiber: 8.1g
- Carbohydrates: 3.9 g
- Protein: 5.1g

83. Coconut Curry Cauliflower Soup

Preparation Time: 15 minutes
Cooking Time: 30 minutes
Servings: 4
Ingredients:

- 1 tbsp. olive oil
- 2-3 tsp. curry powder
- 1 medium onion
- 2 tsp. ground cumin
- 3 garlic cloves
- 1/2 tsp. turmeric powder
- 1 tsp. ginger
- 14 oz. coconut milk
- 14 oz. tomatoes
- 1 cup vegetable broth
- 1 cauliflower
- Salt and pepper

Directions:

1. Take a pot, adds olive oil and onion, and set it on a medium flame for sautéing.
2. After 3 minutes, add garlic, ginger, curry powder, cumin, and turmeric powder and sauté for more than 5 minutes.
3. Now add coconut milk, tomatoes, vegetable broth, and cauliflower and mix it well.
4. Let the mixture heat and bring to boil.
5. Now on low flame, cook it for at least 20 minutes until cauliflower turns into soft, blend the mixture well through a blender and heat the soup for 5 more minutes and add salt and pepper as per taste, serve the hot seasonal soup.

Nutrition:

- Calories: 281
- Fat: 8.1g
- Fiber: 3.8g
- Carbohydrates: 3.2g
- Protein: 4.8g

84. Nutmeg Pumpkin Soup

Preparation Time: 15 minutes
Cooking Time: 20 minutes
Servings: 4
Ingredients:

- 1 tablespoon of butter
- 1 onion (diced)
- 1 16-ounce can of pumpkin puree
- 1 1/3 cups of vegetable broth
- 1/2 tablespoon of nutmeg
- 1/2 tablespoon of sugar
- Salt (to taste)
- Pepper (to taste)
- 3 cups of soymilk or any milk as a substitute

Directions:

1. Using a large saucepan, add onion to margarine and cook it between 3 and 5 minutes until the onion is clear
2. Add pumpkin puree, vegetable broth, sugar, pepper, and other ingredients and stir to combine.
3. Cook in medium heat for between 10 and fifteen minutes
4. Before serving the soup, taste and add more spices, pepper, and salt if necessary
5. Serve soup and enjoy it!

Nutrition:

- Calories: 165
- Fat: 4.9g
- Fiber: 11.9g
- Carbohydrates: 3.5 g
- Protein: 4.2g

85. Thai Coconut Vegetable Soup

Preparation Time: 15 minutes
Cooking Time: 20 minutes
Servings: 4
Ingredients:

- 1 onion (diced)
- 2 bell peppers (red, diced)
- 1/4 teaspoon of cayenne
- 1/2 tablespoon of coriander
- 1/2 tablespoon of cumin
- 4 tablespoons of olive oil
- 1 can of chickpeas
- 1 carrot (sliced)
- 3 garlic cloves
- 1/2 cup of basil or cilantro (fresh chopped)
- 1 teaspoon of salt
- 3 limes (freshly squeezed juice)
- 1/2 cup of vegetable broth
- 1 cup of coconut milk
- 1 cup of peanut butter
- 21/2 cups of tomatoes (finely diced)

Directions:

1. Sauté garlic and onions. Make ingredients to be soft for at least 3 to 5 minutes
2. Leaving out basil, add the rest of the ingredients and allow it to simmer. Cook over low heat for an hour
3. Put the half amount to the food processor, allow it to be very smooth, and return to the pot
4. Add either basil or cilantro, and your coconut food is ready. Before serving the soup, taste and add more seasoning if necessary. Serve, and enjoy!

Nutrition:

- Calories: 151
- Fat: 6.9g
- Fiber: 12.5g
- Carbohydrates: 3.1 g
- Protein: 4.9g

CHAPTER 18:

Dessert Recipes

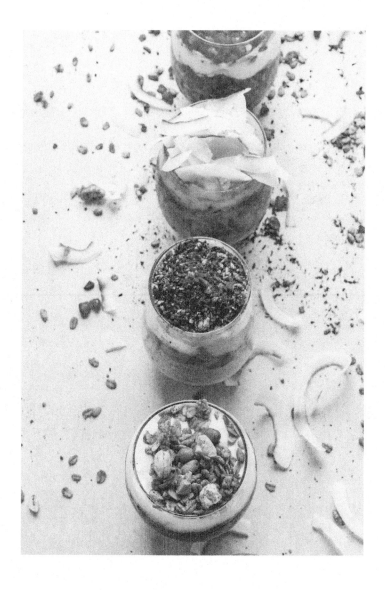

86. Pumpkin Spiced Almonds

Preparation Time: 5 minutes
Cooking Time: 25 minutes
Servings: 4
Ingredients:
- 1 tablespoon olive oil
- 1 ¼ teaspoon pumpkin pie spice
- Pinch salt
- 1 cup whole almonds, raw

Directions:
1. Preheat the oven to 300°F and line a baking sheet with parchment.
2. Whisk together the olive oil, pumpkin pie spice, and salt in a mixing bowl.
3. Toss in the almonds until evenly coated, then spread on the baking sheet.
4. Bake for 25 minutes then cool completely and store in an airtight container.

Nutrition:
- Calories: 170
- Fat: 15.5g
- Protein: 5g
- Carbs: 5.5g
- Fiber: 3g

87. Coco-Macadamia Fat Bombs

Preparation Time: 5 minutes
Cooking Time: None
Servings: 16
Ingredients:

- 1 cup coconut oil
- 1 cup smooth almond butter
- ½ cup unsweetened cocoa powder
- ¼ cup coconut flour
- Liquid stevia extract, to taste
- 16 whole macadamia nuts, raw

Directions:

1. Melt the coconut oil and cashew butter together in a small saucepan.
2. Whisk in the cocoa powder, coconut flour, and liquid stevia to taste.
3. Remove from heat and let cool until it hardens slightly.
4. Divide the mixture into 16 even pieces.
5. Roll each piece into a ball around a macadamia nut and chill until ready to eat.

Nutrition:

- Calories: 255
- Fat: 25.5g
- Protein: 3.5g
- Carbs: 7g
- Fiber: 3g

88. Tzatziki Dip with Cauliflower

Preparation Time: 10 minutes
Cooking Time: None
Servings: 6
Ingredients:

- ½ (8-ounces) package cream cheese, softened
- 1 cup sour cream
- 1 tablespoon ranch seasoning
- 1 English cucumber, diced
- 2 tablespoons chopped chives
- 2 cups cauliflower florets

Directions:

1. Beat the cream cheese with an electric mixer until creamy.
2. Add the sour cream and ranch seasoning, then beat until smooth.
3. Fold in the cucumbers and chives, then chill before serving with cauliflower florets for dipping.

Nutrition:

- Calories: 125
- Fat: 10.5g
- Protein: 10.5g
- Carbs: 5.5g
- Fiber: 1g

89. Curry-Roasted Macadamia Nuts

Preparation Time: 5 minutes
Cooking Time: 25 minutes
Servings: 8
Ingredients:
- 1 ½ tablespoon olive oil
- 1 tablespoon curry powder
- ½ teaspoon salt
- 2 cups macadamia nuts, raw

Directions:
1. Preheat the oven to 300°F and line a baking sheet with parchment.
2. Whisk together the olive oil, curry powder, and salt in a mixing bowl.
3. Toss in the macadamia nuts to coat, then spread on the baking sheet.
4. Bake for 25 minutes until toasted, then cool to room temperature.

Nutrition:
- Calories: 265
- Fat: 28g
- Protein: 3g
- Carbs: 3g
- Fiber: 3g

90. Sesame Almond Fat Bombs
Preparation Time: 5 minutes
Cooking Time: None
Servings: 16
Ingredients:
- 1 cup coconut oil
- 1 cup smooth almond butter
- ½ cup unsweetened cocoa powder
- ¼ cup almond flour
- Liquid stevia extract, to taste
- ½ cup toasted sesame seeds

Directions:
1. Combine the coconut oil and almond butter in a small saucepan.
2. Cook over low heat until melted, then whisk in the cocoa powder, almond flour, and liquid stevia.
3. Remove from heat and let cool until it hardens slightly.
4. Divide the mixture into 16 even pieces and roll into balls.
5. Roll the balls in the toasted sesame seeds and chill until ready to eat.

Nutrition:
- Calories: 260 Fat: 26g Protein: 4g Carbs: 6g Fiber: 2g

91. Coconut Chia Pudding
Preparation Time: 5 minutes
Cooking Time: None
Servings: 6
Ingredients:
- 2 ¼ cup canned coconut milk
- 1 teaspoon vanilla extract
- Pinch salt
- ½ cup chia seeds

Directions:
1. Combine the coconut milk, vanilla, and salt in a bowl.
2. Stir well and sweeten with stevia to taste.
3. Whisk in the chia seeds and chill overnight.
4. Spoon into bowls and serve with chopped nuts or fruit.

Nutrition:
- Calories: 300 Fat: 27.5g Protein: 6g Carbs: 14.5g Fiber: 10g

92. Orange Lime Pudding

Preparation Time: 3 minutes
Cooking Time: 7 minutes
Servings: 4
Ingredients:
- ¼ cup almond milk, unsweetened
- 1 teaspoon agar powder
- ¼ cup coconut cream
- ¼ cup whipping cream
- 1 tablespoon stevia powder
- 1 tablespoon coconut oil

Spices:
- 1 teaspoon orange extract
- 1 teaspoon lime zest, freshly grated

Directions:
1. Plug in your multicooker and place coconut oil in the stainless-steel insert. Press the "Sauté" button and gently stir with a wooden spatula.
2. When melted, add almond milk, coconut cream, and whipping cream. Bring it to a light simmer, stirring constantly.
3. Stir in the stevia powder, agar powder, and orange extract. Cook for another 2-3 minutes, stirring constantly.
4. Turn off the pot and pour the pudding into serving bowls or ramekins immediately.
5. Let it cool to room temperature. Sprinkle with lime zest and refrigerate for 1 hour before serving.

Nutrition:
- Calories: 155
- Fat: 12.3g
- Carbs: 10.7
- Protein: 0.7g
- Fiber: 0.5g

93. Almond Cocoa Spread

Preparation Time: 10 minutes
Cooking Time: 5 minutes
Servings: 3
Ingredients:

- 1 cup almonds
- 2 tablespoons walnuts
- ¼ cup unsweetened cocoa powder
- ¼ cup coconut cream
- 2 tablespoons stevia powder
- 4 tablespoons coconut oil

Spices:

- 1 teaspoon vanilla extract
- ¼ teaspoon nutmeg, ground

Directions:

1. Combine almonds and walnuts in a food processor. Pulse until minced. Add coconut oil and pulse again for 1 minute. Transfer to a large bowl and stir in the stevia powder, vanilla extract, and nutmeg. Set aside.
2. Plug in your multi cooker and pour the coconut cream in the stainless-steel insert. Heat up over the "Sauté" button and then add almond mixture. Stir in the cocoa, nutmeg, and vanilla extract.
3. Cook for 5 minutes, stirring occasionally.
4. Turn off the pot and let it chill to room temperature. Store the spread in an air-tight container or a mason jar.
5. Refrigerate for 20 minutes before serving.
6. Optionally, add some lemon juice for a zesty aroma.

Nutrition:

- Calories: 439
- Fat: 42.9g
- Carbs: 5.4g
- Protein: 9.8g
- Fiber: 7.2g

CHAPTER 19:

Condiments, Sauces and Spreads

94. Taco Seasoning

Preparation Time: 5 minutes
Cooking Time: 5 minutes
Servings: 10
Ingredients:

- 1 tablespoon red chili powder
- 1½ teaspoons ground cumin
- ½ teaspoon paprika
- ¼ teaspoon dried oregano, crushed
- ¼ teaspoon red pepper flakes, crushed
- ¼ teaspoon garlic powder
- ¼ teaspoon onion powder
- Salt and ground black pepper, to taste

Directions:

1. In a bowl, mix together all ingredients.
2. Transfer into an airtight jar to preserve.

Nutrition:

- Calories: 5
- Net Carbs: 0.4g
- Total Fat: 0.2g
- Saturated Fat: 0g
- Cholesterol: 0mg
- Sodium: 24mg
- Total Carbs: 0.8g
- Fiber: 0.4g
- Sugar: 0.1g
- Protein: 0.2g

95. Pumpkin Pie Spice

Preparation Time: 5 minutes
Cooking Time: 5 minutes
Servings: 15
Ingredients:
- 3 tablespoons ground cinnamon
- 2 teaspoons ground nutmeg
- 2 teaspoons ground ginger
- 1½ teaspoons ground allspice
- 1½ teaspoons ground cloves

Directions:
1. In a bowl, mix together all ingredients.
2. Transfer into an airtight jar to preserve.

Nutrition:
- Calories: 7
- Net Carbs: 0.8g
- Total Fat: 0.2g
- Saturated Fat: 0.1g
- Cholesterol: 0mg
- Sodium: 1mg
- Total Carbs: 1.7g
- Fiber: 0.9g
- Sugar: 0.1g
- Protein: 0.1g

96. Garam Masala Powder

Preparation Time: 5 minutes
Cooking Time: 5 minutes
Servings: 10
Ingredients:

- 1 tablespoon ground cumin
- 1 ½ teaspoons ground cardamom
- 1 ½ teaspoons ground coriander
- 1 teaspoon ground cinnamon
- ½ teaspoon ground nutmeg
- ½ teaspoon ground cloves
- 1 ½ teaspoons ground black pepper

Directions:

1. In a bowl, mix together all ingredients.
2. Store in an airtight jar.

Nutrition:

- Calories: 6
- Net Carbs: 0.6g
- Total Fat: 0.2g
- Saturated Fat: 0.1g
- Cholesterol: 0mg
- Sodium: 2mg
- Total Carbs: 1g
- Fiber: 0.4g
- Sugar: 0g
- Protein: 0.2g

97. Poultry Seasoning

Preparation Time: 5 minutes
Cooking Time: 5 minutes
Servings: 10
Ingredients:

- 2 teaspoons dried sage, crushed finely
- 1 teaspoon dried marjoram, crushed finely
- ¾ teaspoon dried rosemary, crushed finely
- 1½ teaspoons dried thyme, crushed finely
- ½ teaspoon ground nutmeg
- ½ teaspoon ground black pepper

Directions:

1. Add all the ingredients in a bowl and stir to combine.
2. Transfer into an airtight jar to preserve.

Nutrition:

- Calories: 2
- Net Carbs: 0.2g
- Total Fat: 0.1g
- Saturated Fat: 0.1g
- Cholesterol: 0mg
- Sodium: 0mg
- Total Carbs: 0.4g
- Fiber: 0.2g
- Sugar: 0g
- Protein: 0.1g

98. Yogurt Tzatziki

Preparation Time: 10 minutes
Cooking Time: 10 minutes
Servings: 12
Ingredients:

- 1 large English cucumber, peeled and grated
- Salt, as required
- 2 cups plain Greek yogurt
- 1 tablespoon fresh lemon juice
- 4 garlic cloves, minced
- 1 tablespoon fresh mint leaves, chopped
- 2 tablespoons fresh dill, chopped
- Pinch of cayenne pepper
- Ground black pepper, as required

Directions:

1. Arrange a colander in the sink.
2. Place the cucumber into the colander and sprinkle with salt.
3. Let it drain for about 10-15 minutes.
4. With your hands, squeeze the cucumber well.
5. Place the cucumber and remaining ingredients in a large bowl and stir to combine.
6. Cover the bowl and place in the refrigerator to chill for at least 4-8 hours before serving.

Nutrition:

- Calories: 36
- Net Carbs: 4.2g
- Total Fat: 0.6g
- Saturated Fat: 0.4g
- Cholesterol: 2mg
- Sodium: 42mg
- Total Carbs: 4.5g
- Fiber: 0.3g
- Sugar: 3.3g
- Protein: 2.7g

99. Basil Pesto

Preparation Time: 10 minutes
Cooking Time: 10 minutes
Servings: 6
Ingredients:

- 2 cups fresh basil
- 4 garlic cloves, peeled
- 2/3 cup Parmesan cheese, grated
- 1/3 cup pine nuts
- ½ cup olive oil
- Salt and ground black pepper, as required

Directions:

1. Place the basil, garlic, Parmesan cheese, and pine nuts in a food processor, and pulse until a chunky mixture is formed.
2. While the motor is running gradually, add the oil and pulse until smooth.
3. Now, add the salt and black pepper, and pulse until well combined.
4. Serve immediately.

Nutrition:

- Calories: 232
- Net Carbs: 1.4g
- Total Fat: 24.2g
- Saturated Fat: 3.8g
- Cholesterol: 7mg
- Sodium: 104mg
- Total Carbs: 1.9g
- Fiber: 0.5g
- Sugar: 0.3g
- Protein: 5g

100. Almond Butter

Preparation Time: 10 minutes
Cooking Time: 15 minutes
Servings: 8
Ingredients:
- 2¼ cups raw almonds
- 1 tablespoon coconut oil
- ¾ teaspoon salt
- 4-6 drops liquid stevia
- ½ teaspoon ground cinnamon

Directions:
1. Preheat your oven to 325°F.
2. Arrange the almonds onto a rimmed baking sheet in an even layer.
3. Bake for about 12-15 minutes.
4. Remove the almonds from the oven and let them cool completely.
5. In a food processor, fitted with metal blade, place the almonds and pulse until a fine meal forms.
6. Add the coconut oil and salt, and pulse for about 6-9 minutes.
7. Add the stevia and cinnamon, and pulse for about 1-2 minutes.
8. You can preserve this almond butter in the refrigerator by placing it into an airtight container.

Nutrition:
- Calories: 170
- Net Carbs: 2.4g
- Total Fat: 15.1g
- Saturated Fat: 2.5g
- Cholesterol: 0mg
- Sodium: 217mg
- Total Carbs: 5.8g
- Fiber: 3.4g
- Sugar: 1.1g
- Protein: 5.7g

101.   Lemon Curd Spread

Preparation Time: 10 minutes
Cooking Time: 10 minutes
Servings: 20
Ingredients:
- 3 large organic eggs
- ½ cup powdered erythritol
- ¼ cup fresh lemon juice
- 2 teaspoons lemon zest, grated
- 4 tablespoons butter, cut into 3 pieces

Directions:
1. In a glass bowl, place the eggs, erythritol, lemon juice, and lemon zest.
2. Arrange the glass bowl over a pan of barely simmering water and soak for about 10 minutes or until the mixture becomes thick, beating continuously.
3. Remove from heat and immediately, stir in the butter.
4. Set aside for about 2-3 minutes.
5. With a wire whisk, beat until smooth and creamy.

Nutrition:
- Calories: 32
- Net Carbs: 0g
- Total Fat: 3.1g
- Saturated Fat: 1.7g
- Cholesterol: 34mg
- Sodium: 27mg
- Total Carbs: 0.2g
- Fiber: 0g
- Sugar: 0.1g
- Protein: 1g

102.   Tahini Spread
Preparation Time: 10 minutes
Cooking Time: 10 minutes
Servings: 4
Ingredients:
- ¼ cup tahini
- 2 garlic cloves, peeled
- 3 tablespoons olive oil
- 3 tablespoons water
- 1½ tablespoons fresh lemon juice
- ¼ teaspoon ground cumin
- Salt and ground black pepper, as required

Directions:
1. Place all of the ingredients in a high-speed blender and pulse until creamy.
2. Pour the smoothie into two glasses and serve immediately.

Nutrition:
- Calories: 183
- Net Carbs: 2.4g
- Total Fat: 18.7g
- Saturated Fat: 2.7g
- Cholesterol: 0mg
- Sodium: 58mg
- Total Carbs: 3.9g
- Fiber: 1.5g
- Sugar: 0.2g
- Protein: 2.7g

CHAPTER 20:

Beverage and Smoothies

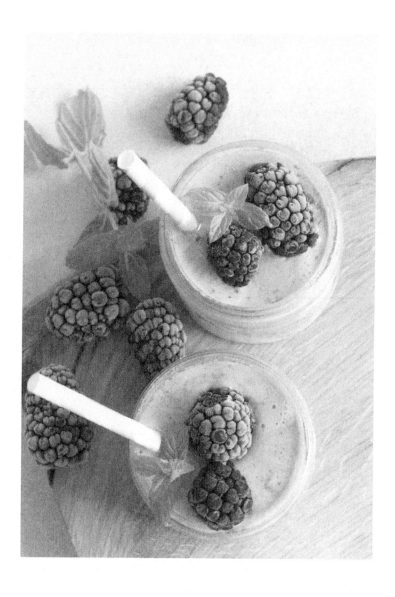

103.   Coconut Smoothie

Preparation Time: 5 minutes
Cooking Time: 0 minutes
Servings: 2
Ingredients:
- 1 cup coconut milk
- 1 cup ice
- 1 banana, sliced
- 2 teaspoons pumpkin pie spice
- ¼ cup pumpkin puree

Directions:
1. In a blender, mix the pumpkin with the rest of the ingredients, pulse, divide into 2 glasses and serve for breakfast.

Nutrition:
- Calories: 100 Fat: 1g
- Fiber: 1g Carbs: 0g
- Protein: 5g

104.   Almond Smoothie

Preparation Time: 10 minutes
Cooking Time: 0 minutes
Servings: 2
Ingredients:
- 1 cup almond milk
- 2 cups spinach
- 1 apple, cored, peeled and cubed
- 1 small ginger piece, grated
- Juice of ½ lime
- 1 orange, peeled and chopped
- 1 cup ice cubes

Directions:
1. In a blender, mix the spinach with the apple and the other ingredients, divide into 2 glasses and serve.

Nutrition:
- Calories: 100 Fat: 2g Fiber: 2g
- Carbs: 6g
- Protein: 8g

105.   Summer Berry Smoothie

Preparation Time: 5 minutes
Cooking Time: 0 minutes
Servings: 4
Ingredients:
- 50g (2ounces) blueberries
- 50g (2ounces) strawberries
- 25g (1ounces) blackcurrants
- 25g (1ounces) red grapes
- 1 carrot, peeled
- 1 orange, peeled
- Juice of 1 lime

Directions:
1. Place all of the ingredients into a blender and cover them with water.
2. Blitz until smooth.
3. You can also add some crushed ice and a mint leaf to garnish.

Nutrition:
- Calories: 186.8 Protein: 16.2g Fat: 1.9g Carbs: 36g

106.   Fruity Parsley Smoothie

Preparation Time: 10 minutes
Cooking Time: 0 minutes
Servings: 3
Ingredients:
- 1 small avocado, peeled and pitted
- 1 cup water
- 2 big bananas, peeled and chopped
- 1 bunch parsley
- 2 pears, peeled, cored and chopped
- 1 cup ice
- 2 plums, pitted
- 1 apple, cored and chopped

Directions:
1. In a blender, mix the avocado with the bananas and the other ingredients, pulse well, divide into glasses and serve.

Nutrition:
- Calories: 120 Fat: 3g Fiber: 4g Carbs: 6g Protein: 9g

107.   Lemony Smoothie

Preparation Time: 10 minutes
Cooking Time: 0 minutes
Servings: 3
Ingredients:
- 2 cups papaya, peeled
- 1 parsley spring
- 1 teaspoon lemon juice
- ½ teaspoon fresh ginger, grated
- 4 ice cubes

Directions:
1. In a blender, mix the papaya with the lemon juice and the other ingredients, pulse and serve.

Nutrition:
- Calories: 90 Fat: 1g
- Fiber: 2g Carbs: 5g Protein: 4g

108.   Orange, Carrot & Kale Smoothie

Preparation Time: 5 minutes
Cooking Time: 0 minutes
Servings: 4
Ingredients:
- 1 carrot, peeled
- 1 orange, peeled
- 1 stick of celery
- 1 apple, cored
- 50g (2ounces) kale
- ½ teaspoon matcha powder

Directions:
1. Place all of the ingredients into a blender and add in enough water to cover them.
2. Process until smooth, serve and enjoy.

Nutrition:
- Calories: 149.9 Fat: 0.9g
- Carbs: 35.6g Protein: 4.1g Fiber: 9.1g

109.   Creamy Strawberry & Cherry Smoothie

Preparation Time: 5 minutes
Cooking Time: 0 minutes
Servings: 4
Ingredients:
- 100g (3½ ounces) strawberries
- 75g (3ounces) frouncesen pitted cherries
- 1 tablespoon plain full-fat yogurt
- 175ml (6fl ounces.) unsweetened soya milk

Directions:
1. Place all of the ingredients into a blender and process until smooth.
2. Serve and enjoy.

Nutrition:
- Calories: 119 Carbs: 21g
- Fat 6g Protein: 2g Fiber: 1g

110.   Lime and Ginger Green Smoothie

Preparation Time: 5 minutes
Cooking Time: 0 minutes
Servings: 1
Ingredients:
- ½ cup dairy free milk
- ½ cup water
- ½ teaspoon fresh ginger
- ½ cup mango chunks
- Juice from 1 lime
- 1 tablespoon dried shredded coconut
- 1 tablespoon flaxseeds
- 1 cup spinach

Directions:
1. Blend together all the ingredients until smooth.
2. Serve and enjoy!

Nutrition:
- Calories: 178 Fat: 1g Carbs: 7g
- Protein: 4g Fiber: 3.5g

111.   Strawberry Spinach Smoothie

Preparation Time: 5 minutes
Cooking Time: 0 minutes
Servings: 1
Ingredients:
- 1 cup whole frouncesen strawberries
- 3 cups packed spinach
- ¼ cup frouncesen pineapple chunks
- 1 medium ripe banana, cut into chunks and frouncesen
- 1 cup unsweetened milk
- 1 tablespoon chia seeds

Directions:
1. Place all the ingredients in a high-powered blender.
2. Blend until smooth.
3. Enjoy!

Nutrition:
- Calories: 266 Fat: 8g
- Carbs: 48g Protein: 9g
- Fiber: 6.3g

112.   Mango & Rocket Arugula Smoothie

Preparation Time: 10 Minutes
Cooking Time: 0 Minutes
Servings: 2
Ingredients:
- 25g (1ounce) fresh rocket arugula
- 150g (5ounces) fresh mango, peeled, de-stoned and chopped
- 1 avocado, de-stoned and peeled
- ½ teaspoon matcha powder
- Juice of 1 lime

Directions:
1. Place all of the ingredients into a blender with enough water to cover them and process until smooth. Add a few ice cubes and enjoy.

Nutrition:
- Calories: 369 Fat: 7.3g
- Carbs: 35g Protein: 18g Fiber: 6.2g

CHAPTER 21:

Snacks

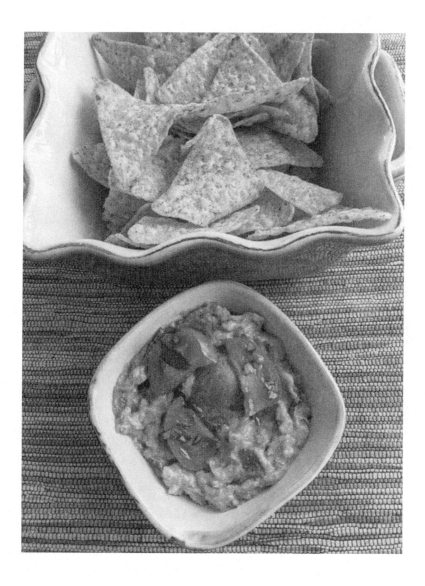

113.   Fried Green Beans Rosemary

Preparation Time: 10 minutes
Cooking Time: 5 minutes
Servings: 2
Ingredients:
- ¾ cup of green beans
- 3 tsp. of minced garlic
- 2 tbsps. of rosemary
- ½ tsp. of salt - 1 tbsp. of butter

Directions:
1. Warm-up an air fryer to 390°F.
2. Put the chopped green beans then brush with butter. Sprinkle salt, minced garlic, and rosemary over then cook within 5 minutes. Serve.

Nutrition:
- Calories: 72 Carbohydrates: 4.5g Fats: 6.3g Protein: 0.7g

114.   Cheesy Cauliflower Croquettes

Preparation Time: 10 minutes
Cooking Time: 16 minutes
Servings: 4
Ingredients:
- 2 cup of cauliflower florets
- 2 tsp. of garlic - ½ cup of onion
- ¾ tsp. of mustard
- ½ tsp. of salt - ½ tsp. of pepper
- 2 tbsps. of butter
- ¾ cup of cheddar cheese

Directions:
1. Microwave the butter. Let it cool.
2. Process the cauliflower florets using a processor. Transfer to a bowl then put chopped onion and cheese.
3. Put minced garlic, mustard, salt, and pepper, then pour melted butter over. Shape the cauliflower batter into medium balls.
4. Warm-up an air fryer to 400°F and cook within 14 minutes. Serve.

Nutrition:
- Calories: 160 Carbohydrates: 5.1g Fats: 13g Protein: 6.8g

115.   Cheesy Mushroom Slices

Preparation Time: 8-10 minutes
Cooking Time: 15 minutes
Servings: 8
Ingredients:

- 2 cup of mushrooms
- 2 eggs
- ¾ cup of almond flour
- ½ cup of cheddar cheese
- 2 tbsps. of butter
- ½ tsp. of pepper
- ¼ tsp. of salt

Directions:

1. Processes chopped mushrooms in a food processor then add eggs, almond flour, and cheddar cheese.
2. Put salt and pepper then pour melted butter into the food processor. Transfer.
3. Warm-up an air fryer to 375°F (191°C).
4. Put the loaf pan on the air fryer's rack then cook within 15 minutes. Slice and serve.

Nutrition:

- Calories: 365
- Carbohydrates: 4.4g
- Fats: 34.6g
- Protein: 10.4g

116. Asparagus Fries

Preparation Time: 10 minutes
Cooking Time: 10 minutes
Servings: 4
Ingredients:

- 10 organic asparagus spears
- 1 tablespoon of organic roasted red pepper
- ¼ cup of almond flour
- ½ teaspoon of garlic powder
- ½ teaspoon of smoked paprika
- 2 tablespoons of parsley
- ½ cup of parmesan cheese, and full-fat
- 2 organic eggs
- 3 tablespoons of mayonnaise, full-fat

Directions:

1. Warm-up oven to 425°F.
2. Process cheese in a food processor, add garlic and parsley, and pulse for 1 minute.
3. Add almond flour, pulse for 30 seconds, transfer, and put paprika.
4. Whisk eggs into a shallow dish.
5. Dip asparagus spears into the egg batter, then coat with parmesan mixture and place it on a baking sheet. Bake in the oven within 10 minutes.
6. Put the mayonnaise in a bowl; add red pepper and whisk, and then chill. Serve with prepared dip.

Nutrition:

- Calories: 453
- Carbohydrates: 5.5g
- Fats: 33.4g
- Protein: 19.1g

117.　　Kale Chips
Preparation Time: 5 minutes
Cooking Time: 12 minutes
Servings: 4
Ingredients:
- 1 organic kale
- 1 tablespoon of salt
- 2 tablespoons of olive oil

Directions:
1. Warm-up oven to 350°F.
2. Put kale leaves into a large plastic bag and add oil. Shake and then spread on a large baking sheet.
3. Bake within 12 minutes. Serve with salt.

Nutrition:
- Calories: 163 Carbohydrates: 14g Fats: 10g Protein: 2g

118.　Guacamole
Preparation Time: 10 minutes
Cooking Time: 0 minutes
Servings: 4
Ingredients:
- 2 organic avocados pitted
- 1/3 organic red onion
- 1 organic jalapeño
- ½ teaspoon of salt
- ½ teaspoon of ground pepper
- 2 tablespoons of tomato salsa
- 1 tablespoon of lime juice
- ½ organic cilantro

Directions:
1. Slice the avocado flesh horizontally and vertically.
2. Mix in onion, jalapeno, and lime juice in a bowl.
3. Put salt and black pepper, add salsa, and mix. Fold in cilantro and serve.

Nutrition:
- Calories: 16.5 Carbohydrates: 0.5g Fats: 1.4g Protein: 0.23g

119.   Zucchini Noodles

Preparation Time: 5 minutes
Cooking Time: 6 minutes
Servings: 2
Ingredients:

- 2 zucchini, spiralized into noodles
- 2 tablespoons of unsalted butter
- 1 ½ tablespoon of garlic
- 3/4 cup of parmesan cheese
- ½ teaspoon of sea salt
- ¼ teaspoon of ground black pepper
- ¼ teaspoon of red chili flakes

Directions:

1. Sauté butter and garlic within 1 minute.
2. Put zucchini noodles, cook within 5 minutes, then put salt and black pepper.
3. Transfer then top with cheese and sprinkle with red chili flakes. Serve.

Nutrition:

- Calories: 298
- Carbohydrates: 2.3g
- Fats: 26.1g
- Fiber: 0.1g
- Protein: 5g

120.   Cauliflower Soufflé

Preparation Time: 10 minutes
Cooking Time: 12 minutes
Servings: 6
Ingredients:

- 1 cauliflower, in florets
- 2 eggs
- 2 tablespoons of heavy cream
- 2 ounces of cream cheese
- ½ cup of sour cream
- ½ cup of asiago cheese
- 1 cup of cheddar cheese
- ¼ cup of chives
- 2 tablespoons of butter, unsalted
- 6 bacon, sugar-free
- 1 cup of water

Directions:

1. Pulse eggs, heavy cream, sour cream, cream cheese, and cheeses in a food processor.
2. Put cauliflower florets, pulse for 2 seconds, and then add butter and chives and pulse for another 2 seconds.
3. Put in water in a pot, and insert a trivet stand.
4. Put the cauliflower batter in a greased round casserole dish then put it on the trivet stand.
5. Cook within 12 minutes at high. Remove, top with bacon, and serve.

Nutrition:

- Calories: 342
- Carbohydrates: 5g
- Fats: 28g
- Protein: 17g

CHAPTER 22:

A Complete 30-Day Meal Plan with Weekly Menu

Week 1

DAYS	BREAKFAST	LUNCH	DINNER
1	Bracing Ginger Smoothie	Cheesy Chicken Cauliflower	Beef-Stuffed Mushrooms
2	Herbed Lamb Chops	Chicken Soup	Rib Roast
3	Nutritious Tuna Patties	Chicken Avocado Salad	Beef Stir Fry
4	Zingy Lemon Fish	Cauliflower Mash	Grilled Pork with Salsa
5	Bacon Avocado Salad	Slow Cooker Chilli	Chicken Pesto
6	Sesame Almond Fat Bombs	Bacon-Wrapped Chicken Bites	Garlic Parmesan Chicken Wings
7	Orange Lime Pudding	Paprika Rubbed Chicken	Crispy Baked Shrimp

Week 2

DAYS	BREAKFAST	LUNCH	DINNER
8	Sesame Keto Bagels	Cheesy Chicken Cauliflower	Beef-Stuffed Mushrooms
9	Spicy Cream Cheese Pancakes	Chicken Soup	Rib Roast
10	Spinach, Mushroom, and Goat Cheese Frittata	Chicken Avocado Salad	Beef Stir Fry
11	Bacon-Wrapped Chicken Bites	Cauliflower Mash	Grilled Pork with Salsa
12	Beans and Sausage	Slow Cooker Chilli	Chicken Pesto
13	Sweet & Sour Pork	Bacon-Wrapped Chicken Bites	Garlic Parmesan Chicken Wings
14	Curry-Roasted Macadamia Nuts	Paprika Rubbed Chicken	Crispy Baked Shrimp

Week 3

DAYS	BREAKFAST	LUNCH	DINNER
15	Paprika Shrimp	Cheesy Chicken Cauliflower	Beef-Stuffed Mushrooms
16	Lime Mackerel	Chicken Soup	Rib Roast
17	Salmon and Lettuce Salad	Chicken Avocado Salad	Beef Stir Fry
18	Cold Green Beans and Avocado Soup	Cauliflower Mash	Grilled Pork with Salsa
19	Healthy Celery Soup	Slow Cooker Chilli	Chicken Pesto
20	Pumpkin Spiced Almonds	Bacon-Wrapped Chicken Bites	Garlic Parmesan Chicken Wings
21	Coco-Macadamia Fat Bombs	Paprika Rubbed Chicken	Crispy Baked Shrimp

Week 4

DAYS	BREAKFAST	LUNCH	DINNER
22	Morning Coconut Porridge	Cheesy Chicken Cauliflower	Beef-Stuffed Mushrooms
23	Bacon Ranch Deviled Eggs	Chicken Soup	Rib Roast
24	Lemony Chicken Drumsticks	Chicken Avocado Salad	Beef-Stuffed Mushrooms
25	Beef and Broccoli Stir-Fry	Cauliflower Mash	Rib Roast
26	Easy Seafood Salad	Cheesy Chicken Cauliflower	Beef Stir Fry
27	Baked Tilapia	Chicken Soup	Grilled Pork with Salsa
28	Paprika Shrimp	Chicken Avocado Salad	Chicken Pesto

Conclusion

Routines ware very important on this diet, and it's something that will help you stay healthy. As such, in this part, we are going to be giving you tips and tricks to make this diet work better for you and help you get an idea of routines that you can put in place for yourself.

Tip number one that is so important is "drink water!" This is absolutely vital for any diet that you're on, and you need it if not on one as well. However, this vital tip is crucial on a keto diet because when you are eating fewer carbs, you are storing less water, meaning that you are going to get dehydrated very easily. You should aim for more than the daily amount of water; however, remember that drinking too much water can be fatal as your kidneys can only handle so much as once. While this has mostly happened to soldiers in the military, it does happen to dieters as well, so it is something to be aware of. Along with that same tip is to keep your electrolytes. You have three major electrolytes in your body. When you are on a keto diet, your body is reducing the amount of water that you store. It can be flushing out the electrolytes that your body needs as well, and this can make you sick. Some of the ways that you can battle this is by either salting your food or drinking bone broth. You can also eat pickled vegetables. Eat when you're hungry instead of snacking or eating constantly. This is also going to help, and when you focus on natural foods and health foods, this will help you even more. Eating foods that are processed is the worst thing you can do for fighting cravings, so you should really get into the routine of trying to eat whole foods instead.

Another routine that you can get into is setting a note somewhere that you can see it that will remind you of why you're doing this in the first place and why it's important to you. Dieting is hard, and you will have moments of weakness where you're wondering why you are doing this. Having a reminder will help you feel better, and it can really help with your perspective.

Tracking progress is something that straddles the fence. A lot of people say that this helps a lot of people and you can celebrate your wins, however, as everyone is different and they have different goals, progress can be slower in some than others. This can cause others to be frustrated and sad, as well as wanting to give up. One of the very most important things to remember is that while progress takes time, and you shouldn't get discouraged if you don't see results right away. With most diets, it takes at least a month to see any results. So, don't get discouraged and keep trying if your body is saying that you can. If you can't, then you will need to talk to your doctor and see if something else is for you.

You should make it a daily or everyday routine to try and lower your stress. Stress will not allow you to get into ketosis, which is that state that keto wants to put you in. The reason for this being that stress increases the hormone known as cortisol in your blood, and it will prevent your body from being able to burn fats for energy. This is because your body has too much sugar in your blood. If you're going through a really high period of stress right now in your life, then this diet is not a great idea. Some great ideas for this would be getting into the habit or routine of taking the time to do something relaxing, like walking and making sure that you're getting enough sleep, leads to the following routine that you need to do.

You need to get enough sleep. This is so important not just for your diet but also for your mind and body as well. Poor sleep also raises those stress hormones that can cause issues for you, so you need to get into the routine of getting seven hours of sleep at night on the minimum and nine hours if you can. If you're getting less than this, you need to change the routine you have in place right now and make sure that you establish a new routine where you are getting more sleep. As a result, your health and diet will be better.

A Short message from the Author:

Hey, are you enjoying the book? I'd love to hear your thoughts!
Many readers do not know how hard reviews are to come by, and how
much they help an author.

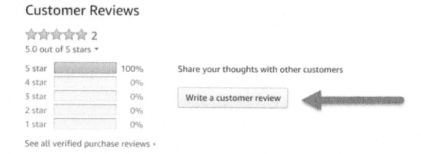

I would be incredibly thankful if you could take just 60 seconds to
write a brief review on Amazon, even if it's just a few sentences!

If you have purchased the paperback version, just going to your
purchases section in Amazon or search this book through Amazon
(Title and Name of the Author) and Click "Write a Review".

Thank you for taking the time to share your thoughts!
Your review will genuinely make a difference for me and help gain
exposure for my work.

Victoria Wills

Printed in Great Britain
by Amazon